# the
# Ostomy Raft

Practical tips for living with an ileostomy or colostomy,

from others in the same boat

## Joan Scott

CAVERHILL PRESS · first edition

*When I woke up in the hospital
I felt like such a dummy
Would I learn to cope?
Should I give up hope?
My ass was on my tummy!!*

*Relax, don't fret, the doctor said
There's nothing you can't do -
You'll work, you'll play
You'll find your way.
And you'll re-learn how to poo!*

*Well, the doc was right. A thousand tips
were mine just for the asking
Now I poop while I sweep
And I poop while I sleep …
I'm the queen of multi-tasking!*

Copyright © 2019 Joan Scott

All rights reserved. Except for the use of quotations in a book review, no part of this book may be reproduced, stored in a retrieval system or database, and/or published in any form or by any electronic or mechanical means, without the prior written permission of the publisher and/or the copyright holder of images.

ISBN 978-1-9990491-0-2

Cover design by Ana Chabrand Design House

The Ostomy Raft

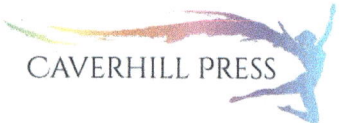

Caverhill Press · First Edition
(caverhillpress@gmail.com)

*Praise for*

# the OSTOMY RAFT

A MUST for anyone who has or is finding they will have to have an ostomy. A plainspeak guide to the realities, challenges and solutions for living with an ostomy. Sprinkled with the author's delightful sense of humor, *the Ostomy Raft* cuts through the taboos of an otherwise sh***y subject with honest and practical knowledge and experience. Joan Scott helps ostomates gain control of their lives ... "Show your ostomy who's boss!!"

**- DIANE WATSON, MSc, Nurse Practitioner (ret)**

Joan has put together some of the best tips available for new and veteran ostomates in this easy-to-follow guide book. I applaud her efforts and commitment to helping others, and I know that many will benefit from her wisdom.

**- ERIC POLSINELLI, VeganOstomy.ca**

After 30 years with an ostomy, I figured I knew it all. Joan's book revealed new tips and tricks that even I hadn't considered. I wish that this book had existed when I was a new ostomate. It is packed full of everything a person living with an ostomy could and should know, and a guide every person coming out of ostomy surgery should have as a resource. Thank you Joan for filling a huge void in the material available for an ostomate. Through books such as *the Ostomy Raft*, information builds much needed advocacy and support that will further educate the world on how so many of us poop and pee differently and that it is perfectly ok!

**- LISA GAUSMAN, Senior Editor, Ostomy Canada magazine**

# Image Credits

**C&S Ostomy Pouch Covers** – http://cspouchcovers.com
    *Ostomy pouch cover (page 55)*

**Cancer Research UK - Creative Commons license**
Original email from CRUK, CC BY-SA 4.0
https://commons.wikimedia.org/w/index.php?curid=34332994
    *Stoma and colostomy bag (page 4)*

**Colo-Magic® Enterprises Ltd.**
    *Bag liner (page 30)*
    *Changing a bag liner (page 41)*

**ConvaTec Inc.**
    *Pre-cut baseplate (page 17)*
    *Cut-to-fit baseplate (page 17)*
    *Moldable baseplate (page 18)*
    *Baseplate with belt tabs (page 21)*
    *Ostomy belt (page 21)*
    *Drainable pouch (page 22)*
    *Closed pouch (page 23)*
    *Adhesive coupling (page 24)*
    *Mechanical coupling (page 24)*
    *Accordion flange (page 25)*
    *Barrier ring (page 32)*
    *Low-pressure adapter (page 35)*

**Heather Scott – Creative Commons license** - Attribution 2.5 Canada, CC BY 2.5 CA
https://www.behance.net/HeatherScottDesigns
This work is licensed under the Creative Commons Attribution 2.5 Canada License. To view a copy of this license, visit http://creativecommons.org/licenses/by/2.5/ca/ or send a letter to Creative Commons, PO Box 1866, Mountain View, CA 94042, USA.
    *Stoma with no hernia (page 125)*
    *Parastomal hernia (page 125)*

**National Institute of Diabetes and Digestive and Kidney Diseases (NIDDK), National Institutes of Health**
    *Small intestine (page 3)*
    *Large intestine (page 3)*

# Image Credits cont'd.

**Salts Healthcare**
    *Stoma collar (page 37)*

**SecuriCare (Medical) Limited**
http.www.securicaremedical.co.uk
    *Emergency kit (page 65)*

**Shutterstock, Inc.**
    *Parts of the colon (page 3)*
    *Colostomy bag – exterior (page 4)*
    *I ♥ my stoma (page 9)*
    *BRAT diet (all images) (page 99)*
    *Pelvic tilt (page 133)*
    *Food Tables (all images) (pages 164-178)*

**wikiHow, Inc.**
    *Baseplate & pouch (page 13)*
    *Ostomy accessories (page 29)*
    *Emptying a drainable pouch (page 39)*
    *Colostomy irrigation (page 46)*

# Prologue

This is a collection of practical tips for ostomates and their caregivers. It's not medical advice – which is best left to professionals. Instead, it's about the realities of day-to-day living with an ostomy. Things I wish I'd known when I started down this path.

The title *"The Ostomy Raft"* is from an allegory I wrote (appears in the Epilogue) about survivors on a raft, helping each other. That's how the book evolved. Some tips are based on personal experience, but a great many more I've learned from others who generously shared their own journeys. They've all made it easier to embrace my "new normal" life. I hope this book will do the same for you.

These are tips primarily for folks with an ileostomy or colostomy. I've had both. But I have no personal experience with a urostomy, so although there may be some overlap, I won't presume to address those specific needs.

Joan Scott

*Medical disclaimer: The information, including text, graphics, and images, are for general educational and information purposes only. It is not intended to be a replacement for professional medical advice, diagnosis or treatment. Always seek the advice of a qualified health care professional with any questions about medical issues or treatment, and never disregard professional medical advice or delay in seeking it because of something you have read in this book.*

*Trademarks: The symbol ® signifies that the indicated trademark is registered and owned by a third party.*

# Contents

**Chapter 1 – IN THE BEGINNING** ..................................................................... 1
   Wrap your head around it ........................................................................ 1
   Understand what's happening ................................................................. 2
   Think like a survivalist ............................................................................. 5
   Set the stage ............................................................................................. 6
   Talk to a stoma nurse ............................................................................... 7
   Talk to others ........................................................................................... 7

**Chapter 2 – THE EARLY DAYS** ........................................................................ 9
   Relax! ......................................................................................................... 9
   Take time to heal ..................................................................................... 10

**Chapter 3 – OSTOMY SUPPLIES** .................................................................... 13
   Choosing an appliance ............................................................................ 14
      1-piece or 2-piece? ........................................................................... 15
   Choosing a baseplate .............................................................................. 17
      1.  Pre-cut, cut-to-fit, or moldable? ................................................ 17
      2.  Flat, convex, or concave? ............................................................ 19
      3.  With or without belt tabs? ........................................................... 20
      4.  Regular or extended wear? ......................................................... 21
   Choosing a pouch .................................................................................... 22
      1.  Drainable or closed/non-drainable? ........................................... 22
      2.  Adhesive or mechanical coupling? .............................................. 24
      3.  Regular or floating/accordion flange? ........................................ 25
      4.  Filters- yay or nay? ...................................................................... 26
      5.  Size – mini, midi or maxi? ............................................................ 27
      6.  Transparent or opaque? ............................................................... 27
   Accessories .............................................................................................. 29

**Chapter 4 – TIME FOR A CHANGE** ............................................................... 39
   Emptying a drainable pouch .................................................................. 39
   Emptying a closed pouch (2-piece appliance) ....................................... 41
   Changing a bag liner (2-piece appliance) .............................................. 41

    Changing your baseplate ................................................................ 42
    Disposal ......................................................................................... 45
    Irrigation ........................................................................................ 46

**Chapter 5 – DAILY LIVING** ........................................................................ 51
    Sleeping ......................................................................................... 51
    Showering & bathing .................................................................... 53
    Dressing ......................................................................................... 54
    Eating & drinking ......................................................................... 55
    Medications ................................................................................... 58
    Getting organized ......................................................................... 59
    Finding support ............................................................................. 61

**Chapter 6 – OUT & ABOUT** ....................................................................... 65
    Emergency kit ................................................................................ 65
    Hospital stays ................................................................................ 68
    Public bathrooms .......................................................................... 68
    Back to work ................................................................................. 69
    Travel ............................................................................................. 72
        Hotels .................................................................................. 73
        Being a houseguest ........................................................... 73
        Air travel ............................................................................. 74
        Road trips or camping ....................................................... 76
    Swimming ..................................................................................... 77

**Chapter 7 – WHAT COULD POSSIBLY GO WRONG?** .................................. 81
    Smells ............................................................................................ 81
    Gas ................................................................................................. 83
    Constipation (colostomies) ........................................................... 87
    Blockages ...................................................................................... 91
    So which is it? – Constipation or blockage? ................................ 95
    Diarrhea ........................................................................................ 97
    Leaks ............................................................................................ 100
    Blowouts ..................................................................................... 106
    Pancaking ................................................................................... 108
    Skin Irritations ............................................................................ 110
       1.   Mechanical irritation ........................................................ 111
       2.   Contact dermatitis ............................................................ 112

  3. Infections ................................................................................................115
  4. Bag just won't stick!................................................................................118
 Stoma issues.......................................................................................................119
 Granulomas ........................................................................................................124
 Hernias ...............................................................................................................125

## FAQs .......................................................................................................................139
 How often should I change my baseplate? ........................................................139
 Sometimes it feels like a bowel movement wants to come out "the old way." Is that normal? .........................................................................................................139
 I still pass something through my rectum sometimes. What's up with that? .........140
 Why does my stoma have two holes? ................................................................141
 What's a Barbie butt? .........................................................................................141
 What can I do to control high output with an ileostomy? ..................................141
 What happens if I need a colonoscopy? .............................................................142
 Is there a trick to using a 'click on' system? I'm hurting myself trying to push the pouch on!......................................................................................................144
 Why can't I get the pouch to stay on when I use a bag liner with a 2-piece 'click & lock' system?..........................................................................................145
 Why is my stool suddenly colored? ....................................................................145
 Should I wear my hernia belt 24/7? ...................................................................146
 What about sex? .................................................................................................146
 Sometimes I feel alone in the world. How many ostomates are out there?............148

## Epilogue – THE OSTOMY RAFT.................................................................................149

## GLOSSARY ...............................................................................................................151

## Appendix A – FOOD TABLES ....................................................................................163
 Gas .....................................................................................................................164
 Constipation .......................................................................................................168
 Food blockages ..................................................................................................173
 Diarrhea..............................................................................................................176

## Appendix B – SYMPTOMS CHECKLIST ....................................................................179

## Appendix C – ILEOSTOMY BLOCKAGE GUIDE........................................................187

## Index ......................................................................................................................191

# Chapter One

# IN THE BEGINNING

*"Knowledge is power and education is your best tool in living well with an ostomy. Ask questions of your healthcare providers and request education from an ostomy specialist before and after surgery ... You can also get information from support groups, online blogs and discussion boards, ostomy manufacturer websites and YouTube."* – **Gwen Spector BSN, RN, COCN, CCP, GI Cancer and Sarcoma Nurse Navigator, Sarah Cannon Cancer Institute at Medical City Plano**

## Wrap your head around it

People end up with an ostomy in different ways.

**A real choice** – There are times when an ostomy can be one of a few medical options available to you and the call is yours. You may be able to try another approach first and leave the ostomy option on the back burner for now. Or after weighing all pros and cons with your physician, you might decide this is the right choice for you.

**Little or no choice** – Because of some disease or disorder, an ostomy is now your best chance at returning to any kind of normal life. Though you may technically still have a choice in the matter, it doesn't feel like that.

**Totally unexpected** – This is usually due to a medical emergency. It could be the result of an accident or some kind of sudden trauma to your body. You might have woken up from surgery to discover that something unexpected happened during the operation, and you now have a bag hanging off your stomach. That kind of thing.

However you got here – whether you had to adjust to the idea of living with an ostomy before or after it happened – it's never easy.

# IN THE BEGINNING

Some people are completely traumatized. Others are immediately grateful that it saved their lives and they begin counting their blessings from Day One. Most of us start off somewhere in between and gradually come to terms with our new reality. That can be helped along with therapy, or medication, or the love and support of others, or the sense of empowerment that comes with learning that you can do this.

What's most important to know is that in the end, the vast majority of people with ostomies learn to accept them and return to as normal a life as possible. And you can too. Just don't beat yourself up about how fast you're getting there. It takes time, and everyone's different. But you'll get there in your own time. Please trust me!

## Understand what's happening

If you're lucky enough to have a heads-up that you're going to have an ostomy, take advantage of that time. Learn a little about ostomies and how to prepare for this change in your life.

Normally, everything you eat or drink is first processed (basically liquified) in your stomach and small intestine. Then it moves into the large intestine (colon), where it's formed into stool and stored in your rectum until it exits your body through the anus.

An ostomy is really just a detour along this route, redirecting the output to come out through a hole in your tummy instead of a hole in your bum. A big difference is that now you can't physically hold it in because there's no sphincter muscle in your abdomen. So it comes out whenever it wants to, and collects in a pouch till you're ready to empty it. Some people "flush out" their colon every day or two in a process called irrigation, instead of relying on a pouch. But more on that later.

There are actually some advantages to having an ostomy if you think about it. You don't have to suffer in silence or worry about soiling yourself if you don't make it to the bathroom in time. You can even poop in the middle of a board meeting or on a long car ride, and no-one will know - except you, sitting there with your secret Mona Lisa smile.

# IN THE BEGINNING

There are two types of bowel-related ostomies:

**Ileostomies** – the ostomy is created somewhere in the **small intestine**. The output exits your body before it ever reaches the large intestine. Output from an ileostomy is usually watery or at least semi-liquid.

–and–

**Colostomies** – the ostomy is created somewhere in the **large intestine** where water and fluids are absorbed by your body, making the output more solid. So output from a colostomy can be pretty much like regular stool. The further along the colon the ostomy is created, the firmer it is.

A little about the anatomy of colostomies: The large intestine starts in your lower right abdomen at the cecum, where it takes over from the small intestine. From there, it goes up (ascending colon), across (transverse colon), down your left side (descending colon), and over (sigmoid colon) to hook up to your rectum. Your colostomy could be located anywhere along this route.

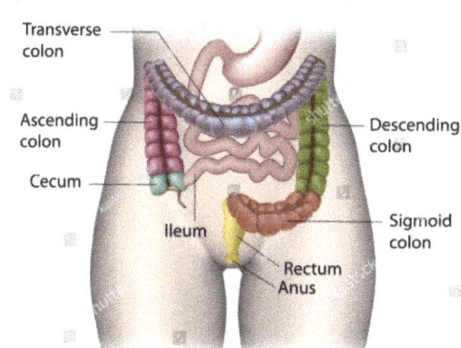

IN THE BEGINNING

You should understand where your own colostomy is located because it makes a difference in whether your stool is more liquid (at the beginning of your large intestine) or more solid (towards the end) – and this affects things like the absorption of medications, transit time (how long it takes food to make its way through your system), and whether or not you might want to consider irrigation later … things that can be very helpful to know at some point. For example, if your colostomy is located near the beginning of the large intestine, it probably functions more like an ileostomy and you should follow those guidelines.

In both ileostomies and colostomies, a small part of your intestine is brought to the surface of your abdomen and protrudes out a little through a hole, called the stoma. That's where your waste comes out and collects in a pouch (which many people call a "colostomy bag," even when it's for an ileostomy).

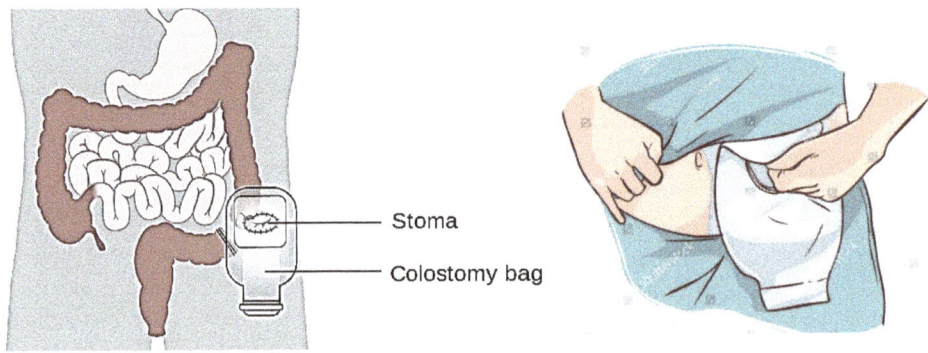

Sometimes, an ostomy is temporary. This might be the case, for example, if you're having some type of surgery involving your bowels or rectum. A temporary ostomy will redirect your output while you heal. After that, everything will be reconnected and you'll be back sitting on the throne with the Sunday paper before you know it.

Other ostomies are for life – for example, if your rectum (at the end of your large intestine, just before the anus) has to be removed due to cancer or other medical problem. Once the rectum is gone, it's gone for good.

IN THE BEGINNING

## Think like a survivalist

Anticipate what you'll need to get through the recovery period, which can be difficult and uncomfortable. Plan ahead to make it as easy as possible.

If you're the cook at home, stock up on supplies like beverages, frozen meals, and canned soups. It'll be a while before you're back on kitchen duty or shopping again.

Will you need someone to walk the dog or drive the kids to school? This is the time to call in favors from friends and loved ones. You'd do it for them, right?

If you have any heavy work to do, do it now. You shouldn't lift anything heavier than 5-10 lbs. (2-5 kilos) for at least a couple of months after surgery.

It's surprising how much everyday items weigh. Here's an example of some things you shouldn't be lifting because they exceed the recommended weight limit:

| *Average weight over 5 lbs./2.5 kg* |
|---|
| Typical woman's purse / briefcase |
| Adult cat |
| Laptop |
| Kettle of water |
| Load of laundry |
| Gallon of milk |
| Bowling ball |

Line up help with housework, like laundry, vacuuming, and changing beds. Anything that involves lifting. You can resume lighter work when you feel up to it, but no heavy housework for a long time.

## IN THE BEGINNING

## Set the stage

When you get home from the hospital, you're going to want to crawl into a freshly made bed that's ready for accidents. Don't tempt fate. Sooner or later you may be very glad you laid down that waterproof mattress pad.

> One woman had a great idea – a dress rehearsal. Before her surgery, she got hold of a sample ostomy pouch and wore it around the house for a few days. She even filled it with water and practiced emptying it. Now that's genius!

Especially in the early days, a roll of paper towels or some hand towels within reach might come in handy too – not just for clean-ups, but also to hold over a leaking pouch on a midnight dash to the bathroom.

You might want to install a bed rail to help you get up without straining your stomach muscles. I used to flop around on the bed like a turtle on its back till I finally installed a rail. What a difference!

If you're having any kind of rectal surgery, particularly if they're closing your rectum, you'll want a cushion to sit on while you're healing. Avoid the "donut hole" or "lifesaver" rings at all cost. They may be great for hemorrhoids, but … well, let's just say that stretching your butt cheeks apart at this point would do more harm than good (cringe!). Instead, use a comfy pillow or folded up blanket, or buy a "waffle cushion" made specially for this purpose. They're square, with multiple holes.

If you're going to have home care nursing for a while, they'll appreciate a clean surface near the bed to lay out supplies and a handy place to dispose of used gauze pads, discarded ostomy products, etc.

Finally, make sure there's a surface in the bathroom to lay out your own supplies for appliance changes. ("Appliance" is the genteel term for what's attached to your stomach). A mirror is essential – so you can see what you're doing, probably while standing or sitting at the toilet. This assumes you're going to be changing your appliance in the bathroom. Most people do, though some prefer to do it while laying on their bed. Whatever works best for you.

## Talk to a stoma nurse

A stoma nurse (AKA wound care nurse or enterostomal therapy/ET nurse) specializes in the care of stomas. Technically, that's the hole in your abdomen – though when most of us say "stoma," we mean the part of your intestine that's poking its little head out.

This nurse will play a key role in your recovery and your life with an ostomy, especially in the first months. He or she will help you decide what supplies you'll need, measure your stoma, teach you how to take care of it, and help you deal with any problems that might come up – like hernias, leaks, and irritated skin.

When ostomy surgery is planned (versus an emergency), a stoma nurse can carefully decide the best location for a stoma on your abdomen and mark the area for the surgeon. The goal is to avoid the waist or any natural crease in your body, and any dips or dimples in the skin – so the appliance will sit flat and be less likely to leak, even when you're bending over. Obviously, there are medical considerations too, and the final decision about placement is the surgeon's. But these practical factors are important and should be taken into consideration.

Ask about a hernia prevention belt, or abdominal binder. The nurse should be able to recommend or even order one for you, and measure you for a good fit. This is particularly important if you have any of the risk factors for what's called a "parastomal hernia," which is quite common after ostomy surgery. Wearing a belt or binder is a minor inconvenience, but better safe than sorry. And better sooner than later. Trust me! See the *What Could Possibly Go Wrong?* chapter for more information on the risks and treatment of hernias.

## Talk to others

Support groups (online, or local groups that meet in person) are a great source of information and encouragement. Some new members haven't had their surgeries yet, or only very recently. Most members have years of experience and knowledge to share. A particular benefit of online groups is that you can ask a question at any time of the day or night and get an answer, usually within minutes, from people who've been there. You can read more about support groups in Chapter 5, *Daily Living*.

## Chapter Two

# THE EARLY DAYS

*I know the struggle of restless nights and a dreary looking recovery ahead. I know the feeling of life being put on hold and the "what now?" questions. I know how difficult it is to depend on other people. I know how frustrating it is to feel like something so simple like walking or going to the bathroom can be taken for granted. I know the "why me?" feeling. But it's just a* blip. *A small blip in your life, and now I'm strong enough to help carry your baggage too. –* **Stacey Willins, IBD Baggage Claim**

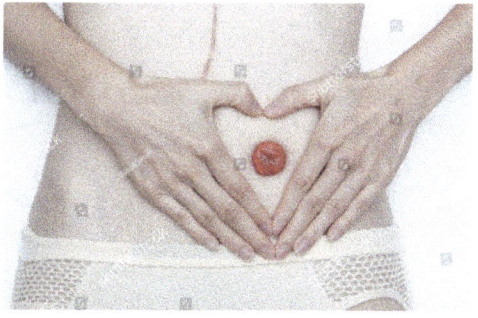

OK, so you made it home and you're starting your new life with an ostomy. Whether it's temporary or permanent, this is the time to make friends with your stoma and learn how to take care of it.

## Relax!

The first hurdle is a mental one. Fear of the unknown. You probably can't imagine how you're going to manage this strange new apparatus, and worry that you'll never feel normal again. Just remember it isn't a race. Take your time. A day, even an hour at a time. You'll get there.

Don't be afraid of your stoma. It isn't fragile. It's pretty much like the inside of your mouth – red, moist, and perfectly okay to touch. There are no nerve endings in the stoma so it won't hurt. And don't worry about "contaminating" it. It spews poop, for Pete's sake!

# THE EARLY DAYS

There *are* a lot of blood vessels near the surface of the stoma, so it's perfectly normal to have a little bleeding if you wipe it, even very gently. But don't be alarmed. It's supposed to do that.

Learn to change your own appliance as soon as you can. The first time can be scary, but you'll feel triumphant afterwards. Have everything you need within reach, then take a breath and go for it. One calm step at a time. Again, this isn't a race. And don't worry about your stoma being exposed while you're fumbling around. It enjoys some fresh air now and then. Just be ready for it to produce a little output without notice. Stomas have a wicked sense of humor.

## Take time to heal

Recovery from any abdominal surgery is a gradual process. Don't rush it, or you might take one step forward and two steps back. Your only job right now is to minimize pain and strain while your body heals.

Don't be a hero! If you have pain, take pain relievers as prescribed. If you let pain get out of control it can be much more difficult to manage.

Avoid any strain on your stomach muscles, which will increase the risk of developing a hernia. You may have been warned not to lift anything heavy for 6 weeks. I'd be even more cautious if I was at a relatively high risk (see the *Hernias* section, Chapter 7, for more on that).

Lifting isn't the only form of strain that can cause a hernia. Chronic coughing, even sneezing, can do it too. Hold a pillow over your abdomen when you cough or sneeze to minimize the strain.

Right after surgery, it may be uncomfortable to lay out flat on a bed. You might find a recliner more comfortable for a while, or propping yourself up on pillows or a bed wedge.

# THE EARLY DAYS

Getting up can be a challenge after any abdominal surgery. In a manual recliner, you could tie a belt around the handle to make it easier to pull. In a bed, many people install a bed rail to grab onto. Some sling a belt or long scarf around their feet, to pull themselves up.

A yoga bench or footstool will make it easier to climb up onto a high bed.

Many people find it difficult to get up from toilets, particularly the low-rise ones. An elevated toilet seat or wall-mounted grab bar can be very helpful.

For a while after surgery, many women with ostomies find it easier to straddle the toilet and pee standing up. I did that. We can't aim as well as men, but it's do-able, and can be WAY more comfortable in the early days!

Bending over can be difficult too. Devices called "retrievers" or "grabbers" are very helpful for picking things up off the floor, and so are long BBQ tongs. Long shoehorns are great. They even make aids for putting on socks. And if you don't normally have pedicures, this is a good time to start. Bending over to clip toenails might be a challenge.

*"When you are new to being an ostomate it is going to feel like all you think about is your ostomy and everything you do is for your ostomy. It may not seem like it at first but it will get better as you live with your ostomy and get used to your new normal."* - **Tn Nahm, *Express Medical Supply***

# Chapter Three

# OSTOMY SUPPLIES

*"Everyone is different and the supplies that work for me may not work for you, and vice versa. I think it's best to try out the many different options and figure out what fits best into your life and what feels the most comfortable."* – Stephanie Hughes, *The Stolen Colon: Living beautifully with an ostomy*

Hopefully, you were sent home from the hospital with enough supplies to last until you can establish your own supply line. Or maybe you have home care nurses who bring their own. But it will soon be on you to manage your own supplies.

Those with private insurance coverage typically place their orders through approved suppliers. Others, including those in countries with national health care, order from suppliers of their choice. The most important thing is to make sure you don't run out. You don't want to be caught duct taping a plastic bag to your stomach until your next order arrives!

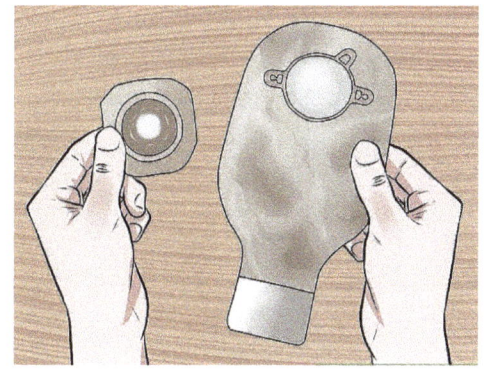

There's a very wide range of ostomy appliances and accessories out there. The basic appliance is a baseplate (AKA wafer, flange, or barrier) that sticks to your skin, and a pouch that attaches to it.

The baseplate has a hole in the middle for your stoma to poke through, so the poo will drop directly into the pouch. Then it's disposed of.

## OSTOMY SUPPLIES

Everyone uses this system at first. Some people with colostomies later switch to irrigation, which uses some different supplies (see the *Irrigation* section in Chapter 4 to learn more about that). But for now, we'll stick to the basics.

Ostomy supplies are constantly evolving, and the needs of individual patients can change too. Every ostomate I know has used different systems and products over the years. So start with the best choices for right now and expect that you'll probably switch to something else down the road.

## Choosing an appliance

Basically, you need to decide what features you want, and whether you want them in a 1-piece or 2-piece system. Anything beyond that, really, is to deal with specific problems that may arise, or to make your life with an ostomy a little easier – the bells & whistles.

> Most suppliers are generous with samples. If you want to try something out, ask for samples. They want your business and welcome a chance to let you try out their products.

There are different brands available. You can get the same types of products from most brands and most suppliers, with slight variations (like different materials or different shapes). So once you know the features and system you want, you can try out a few from different companies to find the ones you like best.

The following pages contain explanations of the many options available in ostomy appliances, followed by a worksheet you can complete to keep your choices straight.

If you find this all too bewildering at first, don't worry about it. The information is here if you want it now, or you can come back to it later when you're ready to learn more. In the meantime, let your stoma nurse decide on the right products for you at this moment and just go with that.

Baseplates

### 1-piece or 2-piece?

This refers to whether the pouch is permanently attached to the baseplate, or separate. Both have their advantages and disadvantages, and most ostomates tend to develop a strong preference for one or the other. Everyone's different and so are their needs.

**1-piece** – the baseplate and pouch are one unit. Every change means changing the whole unit – so it's not a good choice for someone who has to change frequently, because pulling off the baseplate too often can irritate the skin. People who prefer a 1-piece systems often do so because of its simplicity – fewer supplies to manage, less to "fiddle" with, and easier to apply, once you get the hang of it. This kind of appliance also tends to be less expensive than a 2-piece system, and slightly less bulky. Because it's all one piece, the pouch can't pull apart from the baseplate, so many ostomates feel more secure with this type. On the other hand, it also means you can't burp the pouch (to release gas, as described later), or use bag liners (an optional accessory, also described later). And with a 1-piece system, although you can look down and get a birds-eye view of how you're applying it, you can't double check it well from the front, because visibility is hampered or blocked by the pouch. 1-piece appliances usually come in boxes of 5-10.

**2-piece** – the baseplate and pouch are two separate pieces. You remove the pouch to empty it and then reattach it to the baseplate, or discard the pouch and attach new one, as often as needed. Meanwhile, the baseplate stays on you until it's time for a whole appliance change, which is gentler on your skin. It's easier to see what you're doing when applying a 2-piece system. You can check if the hole of the baseplate is placed well around your stoma, if there's too much skin exposed, etc. A 2-piece system offers more versatility. For example, you can rotate the pouch horizontally (to wear under a bathing suit or an ostomy support belt like STEALTH BELT®),

# OSTOMY SUPPLIES

and you can switch between pouches of different sizes – for high output and low output days, or to wear a smaller pouch during the day when you can empty it more frequently, then change to a larger pouch for overnight. You can also use bag liners and burp your pouch with a 2-piece system. One drawback is that if any output has seeped under the baseplate, you won't know about it as quickly as you would with a 1-piece system, because those baseplates are changed more frequently. Also, 2-piece systems tend to be more expensive – but you wear them longer, so it can even out. The baseplates and pouches are ordered separately. Baseplates typically come in boxes of 5-10, and pouches in boxes of 10-20, because you use more of them.

Here's a "cheat sheet" of the pros and cons of both systems, to help you decide which one best fits your individual needs.

## DECISION MATRIX

|  | *1-piece system* | *2-piece system* |
|---|---|---|
| Choices of baseplate/pouch combos | Less choice | More choice ✓ |
| Impact on skin | Less gentle | More gentle ✓ |
| Frequency of baseplate change | More frequent | Less frequent ✓ |
| Checking placement around stoma | Less easy | Easier ✓ |
| Versatility (more pouch choices) | Less versatile | More versatile ✓ |
| Can use bag liners | No | Yes ✓ |
| Can burp pouch | No | Yes ✓ |
| Cost per unit | Less expensive ✓ | More expensive |
| Simplicity | More ✓ | Less |
| Profile | Less bulky ✓ | More bulky |
| Risk of pouch pulling off | No real risk ✓ | Possible |
| Risk of output building up underneath over time, undetected | Less risk ✓ | More risk |

## Choosing a baseplate

The baseplate adheres to your abdomen, with your stoma sticking out through a hole in the middle. When selecting the best baseplate for you, these are the 4 main choices:

1. **Pre-cut, cut-to-fit, or moldable?** (referring to the hole in the middle, which has to be the same size and shape as your stoma)

    **Pre-cut** – These come in a range of standard hole sizes. If you have a nice circular stoma opening, in a common size (diameter), this is a good choice. If the size or shape of your stoma is only slightly different than one of the standard pre-cut holes, you can apply a moldable barrier ring (described later in the *Accessories* section) around the baseplate hole to make up the difference – a sort of retro-fitting. But this means additional time and expense.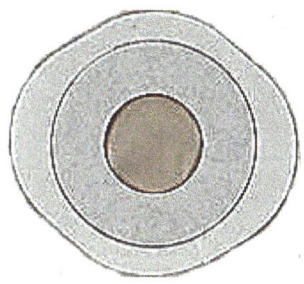

    **Cut-to-fit** – Designed for those with irregularly sized or shaped openings. There's a small starter hole in the middle, but you have to cut your own hole 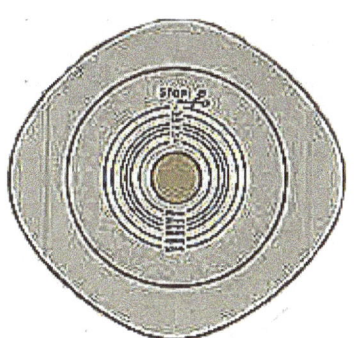 to fit your stoma. Specialized ostomy scissors will make this easier. The baseplates are marked with circular "cut here" guidelines for standard sizes. You'll need to know your exact stoma shape and dimension. If you're in between two sizes, you just cut between those lines. If your opening isn't circular but more irregularly shaped, you or your stoma nurse will have to create a template (on a piece of plastic or cardboard) with a hole that exactly matches your opening, then use a felt pen or marker to trace that shape onto the baseplate, showing where to cut. This isn't the best choice for someone with manual dexterity problems.

# OSTOMY SUPPLIES

**Moldable** – These baseplates have a larger hole, filled with a moldable material around a center opening. There's no cutting or measuring involved here. You stretch or roll up the moldable material until it's roughly the size and shape of your stoma (just a little bigger, actually). After you adhere the baseplate to your abdomen, with your stoma poking through this enlarged opening, you then push the material back to fit snugly around it ("turtlenecking"). This works with stomas of any size or shape. It's a particular advantage to anyone whose stoma dimensions aren't consistent, but sometimes change. One drawback is that the moldable material often swells a little. This can help seal out leaks, but if your stoma is flush or retracted (at or below your skin level), the swelling can cover it too much. Also, moldable baseplates tend to be more expensive than pre-cut or cut-to-fit ones.

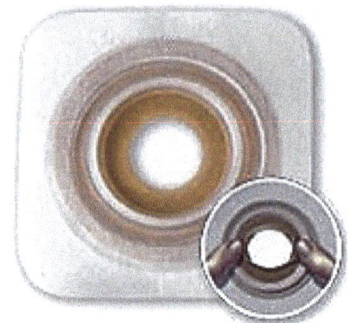

All of these types of baseplates are available for 1-piece and 2-piece systems.

## DECISION MATRIX

|  | *Pre-cut* | *Cut to fit* | *Moldable* |
|---|---|---|---|
| *Stoma = common size, circular* | **Yes** ✓ | Unnecessary | Unnecessary |
| *Stoma = irregular size or shape* | More complicated | **Yes** ✓ | **Yes** ✓ |
| *Stoma changes, inconsistent* | No | **Ok** ✓ | **Best** ✓ |
| *Stoma retracted or flush* | **Yes** ✓ | **Yes** ✓ | No |
| *Manual dexterity problems* | **Yes** ✓ | No | **Yes** ✓ |
| *Cost* | **Less** ✓ | **Less** ✓ | More |

# Baseplates

### 2. Flat, convex, or concave?

**Flat** – These baseplates are flexible, and mold well to your abdomen. They tend to be less expensive than convex or concave baseplates. By default, this is the best choice for most ostomates – particularly if their stomas protrude slightly (which is normal) and they don't have a protruding bulge from a hernia.

**Convex** – This baseplate has a circular, curved, rigid center that sinks down, with a hole in the middle. You press the baseplate down so the stoma protrudes through the hole, then secure it to your abdomen by pressing around the flexible, adhesive edges. It's like a saucer with a hole in the middle and sticky tape under the rim. This is the best choice for an ostomate whose stoma is flush with the skin surface, or retracts below it, which increases the risk of leaking underneath the baseplate or pancaking (output accumulating around the stoma). With the stoma now protruding through the baseplate, the output can drop down more easily into the pouch. You can choose between light, moderate, and deep convexity (referring to how lightly or deeply it presses into your abdomen). Always use the minimum convexity you can, to avoid the risk of pressure sores or ulcers. One drawback of convex baseplates is that since they're more rigid than flat ones, they can be easier to loosen and allow leaks.

**Concave** – These baseplates are designed to adhere well to bulges or protrusions (like hernias) on the abdomen. At this time, they are not available from all manufacturers, but at least one company makes them. The baseplate is flexible and shaped like a flower with five petals that curve downwards, over your bulge. Imagine trying to gift wrap a cantaloupe. It can't be done without creating puckers and creases. That's what it can be like when you try to stick a flat baseplate over a round, protruding hernia bulge. But with a concave baseplate, you place the more sturdy center (with the hole) around the stoma and then press the more flexible "petals" down around the hernia bulge on all sides. There are a

# OSTOMY SUPPLIES

few possible drawbacks, however. They tend to cost a little more than flat baseplates, and there's no convex center to press down around a flush or retracted stoma.

## DECISION MATRIX

|  | Flat | Convex | Concave |
|---:|:---:|:---:|:---:|
| *Flexibility (more secure)* | **More flexible** ✓ | More rigid | **More flexible** ✓ |
| *Cost* | **Less** ✓ | More | More |
| *Protruding stoma* | **Yes** ✓ | No | **Yes** ✓ |
| *Retracted or flush stoma* | No | **Yes** ✓ | No |
| *Bulging hernia* | Maybe | Maybe | **Yes** ✓ |

## 3. With or without belt tabs?

You can order elastic ostomy belts that go around your body and hook onto tabs on both sides of the baseplate or pouch, keeping it snug against your abdomen. (Note: we're not talking about hernia belts here. That's a whole different thing).

This is particularly good for people wearing convex baseplates, because it helps hold them down tightly around the stoma. Ostomates with flat baseplates typically don't need a belt, but might choose to wear one if they're having trouble with their baseplates adhering well, or just want that extra feeling of security. If you're going to wear a belt, be sure to get pouches or baseplates with tabs. Some companies put the tabs on the baseplates, others on the pouches.

# Baseplates

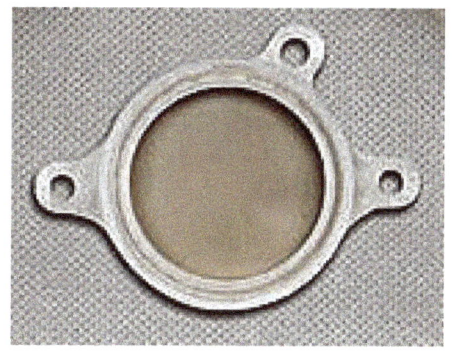

Baseplate with belt tabs

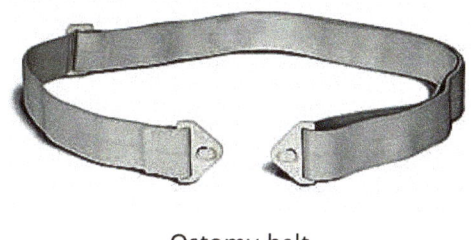

Ostomy belt

The two tabs on the left and right are belt tabs. The tab on the top is just to grab onto, when pulling the pouch off.

## 4. Regular or extended wear?

The most obvious difference between these is that extended wear baseplates can be worn longer than regular wear ones. But there are other factors to consider.

**Regular wear** – The main advantage is that they're less "tacky" and adhesive. They still provide a good seal, but they're gentler on the skin when removing them, particularly if you change baseplates frequently. Because they're less resistant to liquid stool, they're best for colostomates who have firmer, more fully formed stool.

**Extended wear** – These baseplates are a better choice for people with ileostomies, or more liquid stool. They're less likely to allow the liquid to seep under the baseplate and irritate the skin. They tend to cost more than regular wear baseplates, but because they're generally worn longer, it can all even out.

OSTOMY SUPPLIES

**DECISION MATRIX**

|  | *Regular* | *Extended wear* |
|---:|:---:|:---:|
| *Gentle on skin when removing* | More gentle ✓ | Less gentle |
| *Firmer stool* | Yes ✓ | No |
| *Loose/watery stool* | No | Yes ✓ |
| *Wear time* | Shorter | Longer ✓ |

## Choosing a pouch

The pouch attaches to the baseplate. You have 6 basic choices here.

### 1. Drainable or closed/non-drainable?

**Drainable pouches** have an opening at the bottom so you can empty the contents into the toilet, then close it up again and go on your way.

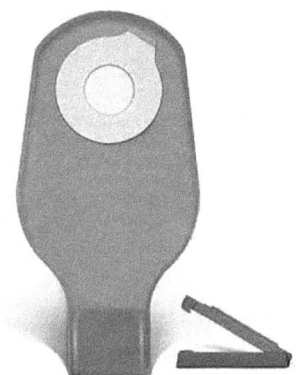

They're good for more liquid stool, which is easier to drain out of the bottom opening and makes it easier to clean the opening afterwards. After emptying, you typically roll up the bottom then close it with either a plastic clip or a VELCRO®-type hook-and-loop fastener. Drainable pouches are more convenient when you're out and about, as you can empty them in a public toilet, close them up again, and you're done. You don't have to worry about disposing of a used pouch.

Drainable pouches can be more cost effective too. Even though they tend to cost more per unit, you can empty and re-use them frequently so they don't have to be changed as often as closed pouches.

**Closed pouches** are not drainable. They're meant to be discarded with the contents and replaced every time. Of course, you can always empty the contents through the stoma hole at the top of the pouch (in a 2-piece system) and re-use it, but that can be pretty messy. Discarding and replacing a closed pouch is a faster process than emptying, cleaning, and resealing a drainable pouch. It's also an easier process for more fully-formed stool, which would have to be squeezed out of a drainable pouch.

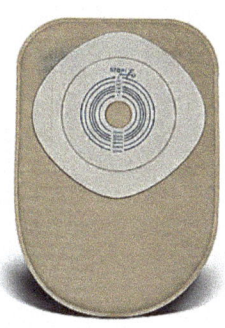

A closed pouch is a good choice for ostomates who use bag liners (in a 2-piece system), and therefore don't need to drain their pouches. You can use liners with either type of pouch, of course, but closed pouches are smaller and simpler. Finally, closed pouches provide more peace of mind for people who worry that the bottom of a drainable pouch might open unexpectedly.

**DECISION MATRIX**

|  | *Drainable* | *Closed* |
|---|---|---|
| *Firmer stool* | Messier | **Tidier** ✓ |
| *Risk of bottom opening* | Slight risk | **N/A** ✓ |
| *Time emptying/changing* | More time | **Less time** ✓ |
| *Using bag liners* | Nothing to drain | **Smaller, simpler** ✓ |
| *Cost per unit* | More costly | **Less costly** ✓ |
| *Cost over time* | **Less costly** ✓ | More costly |
| *Can empty & re-use* | **Yes** ✓ | Not as easily |
| *Convenience in public places* | **More convenient** ✓ | Less convenient |
| *More liquid stool* | **More convenient** ✓ | Less convenient |

OSTOMY SUPPLIES

## 2. Adhesive or mechanical coupling?
This refers to how a pouch attaches to the baseplate in a 2-piece system.

**Adhesive** – Both the pouch and the baseplate have adhesive strips, so the pouch simply sticks on. This is a breeze to do, so it's a great choice for folks with limited manual dexterity. It's also good for anyone concerned about visible bulges under clothing, because it has a very low profile (not bulky). Some people might be nervous that a poop-heavy pouch could fall off (though that's never been a problem in my personal experience). And it's not ideal if you can't see 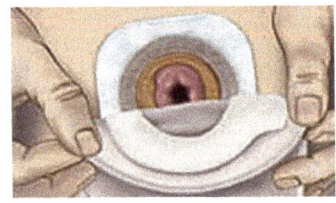 what you're doing, because you generally have to line up the adhesive strips on the pouch with the "landing strips" on the baseplate. You can't use bag liners or burp the pouch (at least not very often), and you can't take the pouch on and off as many times as you can with a mechanical coupling, because at some point the strips will lose their adhesion. This means you'll go through more pouches.

**Mechanical** – This system is bulkier but provides a stronger sense of security that the pouch won't fall off. You either press/snap it onto the rigid protruding ring ("flange") around the hole on the baseplate, or you press it securely onto the flange and then click a locking mechanism that keeps it tight. Because it can be a bit "finicky," at least until you get the hang of it, and requires 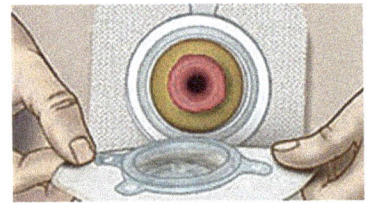 strong pressure from the fingers, it's not the best choice for those with limited manual dexterity or tender abdomens (e.g., if they've just had surgery). It's a good choice for people with limited vision, though, because they can "feel" what they're doing. And it's the only choice for those who want to use bag liners.

## DECISION MATRIX

|  | Adhesive | Mechanical |
|---:|:---:|:---:|
| Profile | Lower/less bulky ✓ | Higher/bulkier |
| Limited manual dexterity | Easier ✓ | More difficult |
| Tender/painful abdomen | Less pressure ✓ | More pressure |
| General ease of use | Easier ✓ | Less easy |
| Sense of security | Lower | Higher ✓ |
| Vision limitations | No | Easier ✓ |
| Frequent burping/emptying | Limited | Unlimited ✓ |
| Can use bag liners | No | Yes ✓ |

## 3. Regular or floating/accordion flange?

The flange is the round, rigid ring on a baseplate that the pouch attaches to in a 2-piece mechanical coupling system. Regular flanges have a pretty low profile. That means you can't slip your fingers under them to help press the pouch on. Instead, you press down hard against the flange (and your abdomen) from the top. But with a floating or accordion flange (pictured), you can slip your fingers under it, so you can grip and squeeze it from the top and bottom. It's a good choice for someone with limited strength or dexterity in their hands or for someone whose abdomen is tender (e.g., following surgery). Some of these flanges have a higher profile, so there might be more of a bulge showing under some clothing. And they tend to be more expensive than regular flanges.

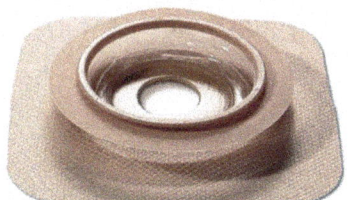

Accordion flange

## OSTOMY SUPPLIES

### DECISION MATRIX

|  | *Regular* | *Floating* |
|---:|---|---|
| *Profile* | Lower/less bulky ✓ | Higher/bulkier |
| *Cost* | Less costly ✓ | More costly |
| *Limited manual dexterity* | More difficult | **Easier** ✓ |
| *Tender/painful abdomen* | More pressure | **Less pressure** ✓ |

### 4. Filters– yay or nay?

Many pouches come with a built-in filter (usually charcoal) that allows gas, but not odors, to pass through. This is so the pouch doesn't inflate like a balloon. There's mixed success with these filters. If they get wet (from the inside or outside), and particularly if they get clogged on the inside, they'll stop working. But if you have a lot of gas, it's better than nothing.

They usually come with adhesive tabs that you can stick over the filter on the outside of the pouch if you want to block it. You might choose to do this if you're not particularly concerned with gas building up, but more concerned about keeping a little air or space inside the pouch for your output to drop into.

So it really comes down to being sure to order baseplates with a filter if gas buildup is a concern, and just covering up the filter if you don't need it – since most pouches come with the filter anyway.

## 5. Size - mini, midi or maxi?

Pouches are available in a range of sizes, holding different volumes of output. And you can get them in different sizes to fit the same baseplate.

After your body has adjusted to your ostomy, you'll probably settle into a predictable rhythm and volume of output and get to know what size pouch is best for you normally. Probably a regular, or midi size, for most of us.

People with higher output stomas often wear large or extra-large pouches every day, or at least overnight, so they can sleep with less interruption.

You may want to wear a small pouch temporarily, like for swimming or having sex, particularly if you expect to have little or no output during that time.

And ostomates who irrigate regularly might only need a small or even micro-sized pouch most or all of the time.

After you've established your regular size, you might want to have a few samples of other sizes stashed away, in case the need arises.

## 6. Transparent or opaque?

This simply refers to whether or not you want to be able to see what's happening inside your pouch. If so, order pouches that are clear or transparent. If you don't care about seeing inside, order opaque pouches. That means they're covered in a light material you can't see through – usually beige. They often have a flap that you can lift up to see the stoma area if the need arises, though, through a transparent window. Both are easy to come by. All or almost all brands carry both clear and opaque pouches.

OSTOMY SUPPLIES

## **WORKSHEET**

You can complete this worksheet to keep track of your choices, then record the product numbers that fit your needs underneath it. If you're using a 2-piece appliance, be sure to order the baseplates and pouches from the same manufacturer, so they fit together. Most manufacturers have toll-free numbers where you can call to discuss the products they have that meet your needs.

| Type | ☐ 1-piece | ☐ 2-piece | |
|---|---|---|---|
| **Baseplate** | ☐ Pre-cut | ☐ Cut-to-fit | ☐ Moldable |
| | ☐ Flat | ☐ Convex | ☐ Concave |
| | ☐ Belt tabs | ☐ No belt tabs | |
| | ☐ Regular wear | ☐ Extended wear | |
| **Pouch** | ☐ Drainable | ☐ Closed | |
| | ☐ Adhesive | ☐ Mechanical | |
| | ☐ Regular flange | ☐ Floating flange | |
| | ☐ Filter | ☐ Not necessary | |
| | ☐ Mini | ☐ Midi/regular | ☐ Maxi |
| | ☐ Transparent | ☐ Opaque | |

Manufacturer: _____

1-piece: Product # _____

2-piece: ⎧ Baseplates: Product # _____
⎩ Pouches: Product # _____

Stoma size: _____

# Accessories

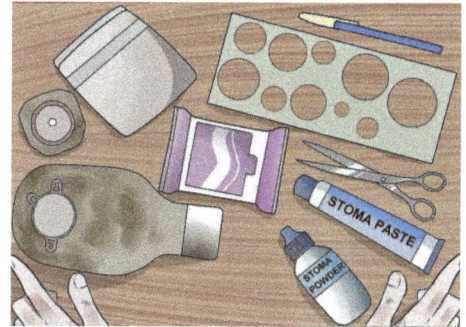

All these products are available from most ostomy suppliers. If you're new to ostomies, you don't need to worry about learning about all of them now. You may never need some or even any of them. The descriptions are just here for you to consult as needed.

## Adhesive removers

Baseplates are made with special adhesives to (hopefully) stick tightly to your skin for days. But of course they're not going to suddenly pull away easily just because it's time to change them. That's why you have to be gentle when removing them. If you need a little help, adhesive removers are there for you.

They usually come in wipes, in individual sealed packets, or as a spray. In both cases, apply the remover as you work around the baseplate, gently removing it.

You can also use it to remove any residue left on the skin from the baseplate or from products like paste, strips, or rings. Even if you can't see it, you can tell there's residue left behind if your skin feels tacky. This residue can usually come off with a little soap and water too, but an adhesive remover works well if you need a little extra cleaning power.

Because the remover breaks down adhesive, you definitely don't want any trace of it left behind on your skin when you apply a new baseplate. Make sure you rinse or wash it off well after it's done its job, then let your skin dry completely, and you're good to go.

## OSTOMY SUPPLIES

### Bag liners

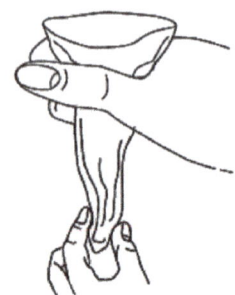

These are small plastic bags, much like doggie bags, that you insert down into your pouch. When you have output to empty, you simply pull the bag liner out, dispose of it (with its contents), pop in a new liner, and go on with your day.

They really work best for colostomates, though I've heard of a few ileostomates using them successfully too. You don't *need* to use them. They're entirely optional. Many people (like me) love them. Others don't.

The liners are supposedly flushable, and some claim to be decomposable. See the *Time for a Change* chapter for more detailed instructions on how to use them. One drawback is that they're definitely not flushable if you have a septic system, and you'd want to be careful if your regular plumbing blocks easily. As ostomates, we can all relate to that, right?

> Even if you don't have a septic system, many sources say anything but human waste and toilet paper will eventually clog up the system. You can always dispose of used bag liners in a sealed plastic bag if you want to play it safe.

There are several benefits to using liners. It's a quick, tidy process. No smears to deal with, no washing out a pouch, no poopy fingers. They're way less expensive than pouches (just pennies each), and you'll go through far fewer pouches this way because they don't get soiled at all.

Bag liners generally come in two sizes, to accommodate different size stoma holes. They work with most sizes, but if your baseplate hole is unusually small, this probably isn't a good choice, particularly if you have a colostomy. You'd have trouble pulling out a bagful of firm stool through such a small opening.

Bag liners can be used with either drainable or closed pouches, although there's actually no need for a drainable pouch with a bag liner.

They work with almost all 2-piece systems with a mechanical coupling. There may be a few brands they don't work with because of the way the coupling system is designed. So try a sample first to make sure it works with your appliance.

They don't work at all with 1-piece systems or 2-piece self-adhesive types, because the plastic liner protrudes outside the rim of the hole in the pouch and this would interfere with adhesion (of the 1-piece baseplate to your skin, or of the adhesive pouch to your 2-piece baseplate).

## Barrier paste or strips

Also called stoma paste, this isn't actually a paste in the sense of being an adhesive. It's more like caulking. Or if you're a golfer, it's like something to fill in divots. Basically, the paste is used to fill any gaps between your skin and the baseplate, to prevent leaking.

Paste can come in a tube, that you squeeze out, or in strips, where you tear off pieces as needed.

If you have dips, indentations, or any other irregularities around the stoma, use the paste to fill them in and create a smooth, flat surface before applying the baseplate.

If you don't have one or two particular crevices, but find that the skin surface around the stoma is just generally uneven, you can apply a ring of paste around the edge of your stoma hole, or around the hole on the baseplate.

It doesn't matter if you apply the paste to your skin or to the baseplate.

In either case, allow it to set for a minute or two before applying the baseplate to your skin.

Some pastes contain alcohol. Others have a low alcohol content or even none. The alcohol might cause a brief burning or stinging sensation. That's normal. But if it's more than that, or if you suspect you're allergic to it, switch to an alcohol-free brand.

Always use the minimum amount of paste needed. Remember – less is more. Don't use paste, or any other ostomy product for that matter, if you don't need to.

## Barrier rings

Some people use these flat, pliable rings to encircle the stoma (or the hole in your baseplate) and help prevent leaks by absorbing moisture. This makes them swell a little, so they tend to break down and require a baseplate change more quickly. This is sometimes called "melting." Different brands last longer than others, so try out a few samples to find the one that works best for you.

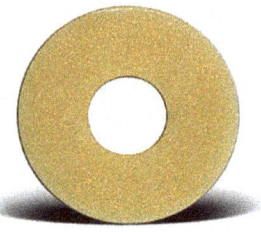

Like with barrier paste, you can apply it directly to your skin, completely encircling your stoma, or you can put it on the underside of the baseplate first, all around the hole, and then apply the baseplate to the skin.

It can also be used to "retrofit" the baseplate opening. For example, if your stoma isn't a true circle, but more of an oval or irregular shape, you can use a baseplate with a pre-cut circular hole that's a little too big. Make sure it exposes your entire stoma. Now cut off a piece of a barrier ring, warm it in your hand to make it even more pliable, and mold or flatten it to the shape you need. Place it along the edge of the hole of the baseplate where any skin would be exposed. Hold the baseplate over your stoma to make sure it's an exact fit. If not, adjust the barrier ring material till you're satisfied. Then apply the baseplate to your skin.

Similarly, if your stoma opening is round but in between two hole sizes of pre-cut baseplates, you can use the bigger size and apply a piece of barrier ring all around the hole, "downsizing" it to fit you exactly.

You can also use a piece of a barrier ring to fill in gaps underneath the baseplate, between your skin and the baseplate, the same way you'd use barrier paste.

Keep in mind that these rings are to be used only if and when you're experiencing leaks. Otherwise, don't use them preventatively. Baseplates are designed to stick best to clean, dry skin, with no other products. It bears repeating – don't use any product, including barrier paste or barrier rings, if you don't need to.

**Barrier sheets** (also called skin barrier sheets, or protective sheets)

These are thin, flexible, adhesive sheets (usually square and transparent) that provide a protective layer between your skin and the baseplate. They're typically used to protect irritated skin.

Cut a hole in the sheet to match your stoma, then apply it over the stoma and surrounding skin (which should be clean and dry). Then apply your baseplate on top of the sheet.

If you use pre-cut baseplates, use one as a template to cut the hole in the sheet. Otherwise, use the templates that typically come with baseplates or create your own, to match the size and shape of your stoma opening.

You don't need to use the whole barrier sheet. You can cut a piece to cover only a smaller area that is irritated.

There are barrier sheets specifically marketed for use with ostomies, but you can also use other hydrocolloid dressings that are designed for wound protection generally. Two common brands are DUODERM® and TEGADERM®. They can come in square sheets or in rolls, which you cut to the size and shape you need.

Barrier sheets are good for temporary use, to allow irritated skin to heal or to buy time while you're searching for a product you don't react to. If you find you need to use them permanently, you should talk to a stoma nurse to investigate why this is happening and what else you can do about it.

**Barrier sprays or wipes**

These products (also called skin barriers or skin sealants) are sprayed or dabbed onto the skin around your stoma to form an invisible barrier between the skin and the baseplate, like barrier sheets do. Whether the protective product was applied on your skin by a spray or wipe, always let it dry thoroughly before applying the baseplate

They're not necessary if your skin is healthy under there. You should always follow the less-is-more rule. However …

- If there's any irritation, it can help to protect the skin while it heals.
- If the skin is fragile and easily irritated by frequent changes of the baseplate, it provides a layer of protection.
- It's good for allergies to adhesives, providing a protective layer between the skin and baseplate.
- It's also used to seal in any other products you may have used (stoma powder, for example) that might interfere with adhesion.

**Baseplate adhesives** (also called medical adhesives or ostomy adhesives)

These come in different forms - wipes, sprays, liquids, etc. Baseplates have an adhesive backing of their own, of course. But these additional adhesives are for ostomates who are still having trouble getting their baseplates to stick. You generally apply the adhesive to your skin, or to the back of the baseplate. Follow the product's instructions for any specific techniques. For example, you may need to wait until it becomes tacky.

# Accessories

## Flange extenders

These are adhesive tapes or strips that are usually C-shaped or Y-shaped, and are applied around the outside edges of the baseplate, like a picture frame, to increase adhesion to your abdomen. You can cut them if you only need extra adhesion in one place.

## Floating or accordion flanges

In the post-surgery period, pressing down hard on your abdomen can be painful, even traumatic to your wound. You can get around this by using a floating or accordion flange, as described on page 25. These serve the same purpose as low-pressure adapters (below) - letting you slip some fingers under the flange to help attach the pouch. The difference is that floating or accordion flanges are a built-in feature of the baseplate, not a separate piece.

## Low-pressure adapter

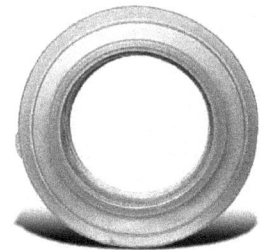

This is a circular device, pictured at right, that you place between the baseplate and the pouch, providing a gap for you to "squeeze-press" the pouch on with your fingers instead of pressing down on your abdomen.

## Lubricating deodorant

This product comes in a squeeze bottle. You squirt a little into the pouch (or bag liner) every time you empty or change it. It's designed to deodorize the contents of the pouch, and lubricate it so your output will slide down to the bottom more easily, rather than pancaking around your stoma. You might like the scent of one brand more than another so try out a few before deciding.

# OSTOMY SUPPLIES

### Ostomy scissors

Specialized ostomy scissors are designed to cut stoma holes in baseplates. They're curved or angled, with blunt tips, and are available from many ostomy supply companies. There are cheap ones available, but they don't cut well for very long. If you're going to be cutting your own holes for the foreseeable future, try to get the best scissors you can. This is a case where you get what you pay for.

### Stoma bridges

Stoma bridges are designed to prevent pancaking. They're not available everywhere. At this time, you can get them in the UK, and hopefully they'll expand to other countries. The bridges are small foam-like cubes with an adhesive backing on one side. You remove the protective cover from that side and stick it inside the pouch in the area of your stoma. You can use one or more at a time (like one above the stoma, or one on each side of it). The idea is that it creates a gap between the front and back of the pouch, preventing the pouch from sticking to itself and allowing output to drop down. *(Note: a "stoma bridge" is also the name of a surgical product or technique, but that's not what we're talking about here).*

### Stoma caps

These are very small, closed pouches often worn by people who irrigate, and whose output is predictable and well regulated. They're worn in between irrigations, and are really more like caps than pouches. Some ostomates who don't irrigate also use them to cover their stomas for brief periods, like swimming or intimate moments, when they want to minimize the size of their appliance and are pretty sure there won't be much output for the next little while.

## Stoma collars

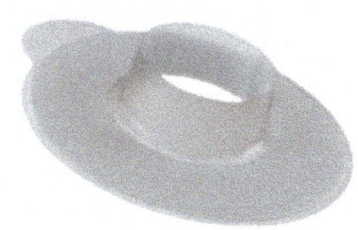

Also called "stoma hats," because they're like a wide-brimmed hat with the top cut off. These are round adhesive disks with a spout-shaped cylindrical collar in the middle that fits around the stoma. They're adhered to the skin before applying the baseplate and are designed to prevent output from leaking under the baseplate by encouraging the output to flow through the spout and drop directly into the pouch.

## Stoma guards

Also called "stoma protectors," these are like athletic cups for stomas – rigid devices that literally guard your stoma from injury. They're designed to be worn during sports, or in any situation where an ostomate might suffer a direct impact to the stoma. Depending on the location of your stoma, they can also be helpful to prevent pant belts or seatbelts from pressing directly on it. There are many versions on the market. Most are held in place by a type of belt.

## Stoma powder

If the little perimeter of skin that circles the stoma is exposed to watery or damp output, it can become irritated. Stoma powder is specially made to absorb moisture on the skin surrounding the stoma (not all the skin under your baseplate).

> You can substitute regular products found around the home for many ostomy products. But stoma powder isn't one of them! Talcum powder, corn starch ... none of these would help and might even cause more problems.

## OSTOMY SUPPLIES

Stoma powder isn't medicated. It isn't intended to heal the skin, but just to keep it dry while it heals by itself.

It's meant to be used only when the skin circling the stoma is occasionally irritated, not all the time. If the edge of your stoma opening is always red, raw, and irritated, then you need to address that issue. Using powder with every baseplate change won't solve the problem.

Make sure your skin is clean and dry before using the powder.

The powder can be applied in different ways. It comes in a "puff" bottle, so it's often puffed onto the skin, circling around the stoma. The less-is-more rule applies here. You don't want a thick build-up of powder, just a thin layer. So you should brush off any excess (whatever doesn't stick to the raw edge of the skin), with a soft tissue. A clean, soft makeup brush works well too.

Another way to apply the powder is to puff some along the side of your index finger, using another finger to push it into a line. Then press the line onto your skin and around your stoma with the index finger. Again, brush off any excess.

If you feel you need more, you can apply 2-3 thin layers of powder (versus one thick one), with a layer of a skin barrier product in between, allowing it to thoroughly dry before applying the next layer of powder. This is called "crusting."

# Chapter Four

## TIME FOR A CHANGE

---

*"Let's face it, we aren't born knowing how to change an ostomy appliance or how to handle leaks, and it can be overwhelming at first. Learning how to change an appliance properly can give you the confidence in knowing that it'll be secure and reliable."* - **Eric Polsinelli, VeganOstomy.ca**

Here's a rundown of the standard procedures for emptying your pouch or changing the whole appliance. These are the basics.

### Emptying a drainable pouch

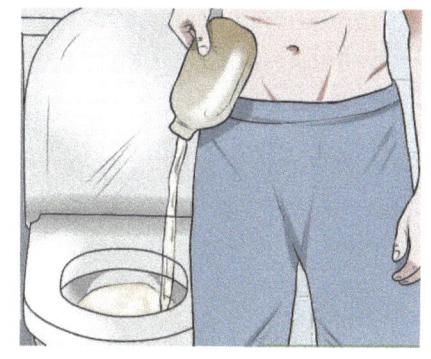

You should empty your pouch when it's about 1/3 full. You can wait till it's 1/2 full but don't push it much past that or you'll risk it suddenly filling up - which can have some unpleasant consequences.

Open the bottom and empty the contents into the toilet. If your output is semi-soft, you can squeeze it out like toothpaste. If it's more watery (common with ileostomies), it'll pour out easily … unless the pouch is so full and gassy that it's about to burst. In that case, as soon as you open the bottom it might start spraying around the room like an out-of-control firehose! If you think this might happen, get as low down to the toilet as you can, and take careful aim. Expect a gusher. And make a mental note to try not to let so much gas build up in your pouch again.

TIME FOR A CHANGE

> To prevent splash backs, lay a few squares of toilet paper on the water before emptying your pouch.

Some people empty their pouches between their legs while sitting on the toilet. Others stand up at the toilet, or sit on a chair facing it. Whatever works best for you.

After emptying, wipe the opening at the bottom of the pouch with toilet paper. Some folks use a squeeze bottle to squirt warm water into the opening and swish it around in the pouch first.

Most people re-use the pouch a few times, particularly if it isn't too soiled, before changing to a fresh one. If you're wearing a 2-piece appliance, you'll probably change your pouch more often than your baseplate.

Some ostomates wash out their pouch really thoroughly, changing to a new pouch so the old one can air dry before being re-used. I know that a few nurses have recommended against this, but if you're the kind of person who cringes at the very thought of wearing a pouch that's "smeared" inside, you can try it. The most important thing is for you to be comfortable and at ease.

The bottoms of drainable pouches typically come with a plastic clip or a VELCRO® hook-and-loop type flap that rolls up and seals the pouch shut. Both good. Just remember to seal it up when you're done. If you forget to close the bottom of the pouch, you'll find out about it soon enough. Yuck! But take heart. We've all been there. It's a lesson you only have to learn once. Twice at the most.

> For peace of mind, some people put one of those black binder clips from office supply stores on the bottom of their sealed drainable pouch, to make extra sure it won't open accidentally.

# TIME FOR A CHANGE

## Emptying a closed pouch (2-piece appliance)

You should do this when it's 1/3 or 1/2 full, the same as a drainable pouch. The only difference is that if you're going to empty and re-use the pouch, you empty it from the hole that goes over your stoma, instead of from the bottom. Again, you can rinse it out and re-use it, or toss it out and put on a fresh one.

## Changing a bag liner (2-piece appliance)

This is as simple as it gets. When it's time to empty, simply pull the liner out of the hole in the pouch and dispose of it. The pouch itself remains unsoiled.

Bag liners are supposed to be flushable, except in a septic system. But if it's particularly full of solid stool, squeeze the contents out into the toilet first. Otherwise, it can be like trying to flush a brick.

Many people say you should never flush anything but toilet paper. If you're hesitant to flush the bag liner, you can dispose of the empty liner as you do a used pouch. This is what I do. I keep my used, empty liners in a resealable plastic bag until trash day.

To put a new liner in the pouch, just push it in then insert a couple of fingers down as far as you can and wriggle them around to open it up a bit inside. You can also blow into it. Leave some of the liner sticking out, all around the hole. You don't have to be fanatic about smoothing it out. It will never be neat & tidy. Just be sure you leave enough sticking out to "catch" all the way around the hole when you click or press the pouch back onto the baseplate.

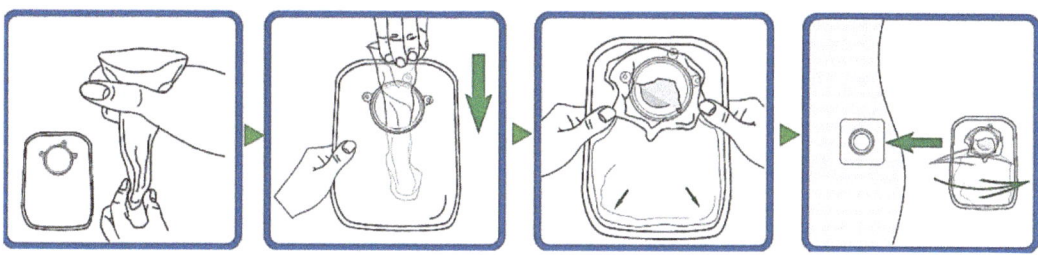

TIME FOR A CHANGE

## Changing your baseplate

There's no one-size-fits-all schedule for this. Everyone's different. It's mostly about avoiding leaks (which are obvious) or slow seepages under the baseplate (which can be sneakier). As soon as any output gets under there, you need to change the baseplate.

That doesn't mean you should wait for a leak before changing. Hopefully, there's no leak. But to avoid skin problems, you need to take the baseplate off, clean your skin, and put on a new one, on a regular basis.

Some people have to change their appliance several times a day (usually because of problems with leaking). Others can go a week or even longer. Most people are somewhere in between. Over time, you'll get to know what's average for you.

> If you tend to go several days between changes, it's easy to lose track of how long you've been wearing the same baseplate. In that case, every time you change your baseplate, you should write the day of the week on the outside of the pouch with a permanent marker.

### Step 1 – Remove appliance

You might find it easiest to do the change standing, or sitting, or lying down. Whatever works for you. I stand at the toilet, in case there's any output while my stoma's exposed. Those who sit or lie down usually have gauze or tissue ready to place over their stomas to catch any leaks.

The first step is to remove the baseplate (with or without an attached pouch). Don't just rip it off like a bandage. Use one hand to hold or stretch your skin while the other hand gently pulls off the baseplate, working your way around it.

If your skin is fragile or if you feel the baseplate is sticking a little too well, you can use an adhesive remover around the edge (they usually come as individually wrapped wipes), one small area at a time, gently pulling the baseplate off your skin as you go.

> Have everything you'll need within reach. You don't want to take off your baseplate, then realize you have to walk across the bathroom to grab something. Believe me, that's exactly when your stoma will decide to wake up!

If there's a build-up of adhesive on your skin after you've removed the baseplate, take it off with another adhesive remover wipe. You'll know if you need to do this because your skin will feel tacky or you'll actually see or feel little clumps of adhesive build-up.

## Step 2 – Wash the area

Next, gently wash the skin around the stoma. Don't scrub, but be thorough. Most stoma nurses say it's best to use a soft cloth and warm water. No soap. If you feel you really must use soap, the milder the better. Avoid anything with perfume, oils, or deodorant.

I used to use baby washcloths, particularly when my skin was irritated, but now that the area's healthy I use a good quality, soft paper towel. Don't actually wash the stoma itself, just the skin around it that's been covered by the baseplate.

If you've used soap or any other kind of product, like adhesive remover, make sure you rinse really well.

# TIME FOR A CHANGE

It's perfectly ok to get some soap or water on the stoma. Some people even take baths with their stomas exposed. Just make sure to rinse thoroughly afterwards.

You may need to put some products on your skin or baseplate at this point, depending on your individual situation. These are described later in the *What Could Possibly Go Wrong?* chapter.

Make sure the area is bone dry after rinsing or applying any products. You can let your skin air dry, or use a blow dryer on a gentle setting.

## Step 3 – apply the new baseplate

Typically, there's a flimsy backing on the baseplate that keeps the adhesive side sticky and clean. Peel it off, then apply the baseplate over your stoma, making sure very little or no skin is exposed around edge of the stoma and visible through the hole. It should be a pretty exact fit.

Some ostomates and nurses say there can or even should be a very tiny circle of skin visible around the stoma (a maximum of 1/8" or .33 cm). This is to be extra sure that your stoma opening doesn't extend beneath the baseplate, which could result in leaking.

It's really up to you. If you find that leaving any skin exposed at all makes it red and irritated, then try an exact fit. If you find an exact fit leads to leaking or seepage under the baseplate, try leaving a small circle of skin visible. Over time, you'll get to know what works best for you.

Some ostomates gently warm the baseplate for a few minutes with a hair dryer before applying it. This can make the baseplate adhere better to your skin. It isn't a must-do step for everyone, but if you find you need some extra adhesion, it's something to try.

Once the baseplate is on, make sure it's secure by pressing firmly all around it, taking special care to press the circular area immediately around the stoma with your finger.

With a 1-piece appliance, you're good to go. Otherwise, the next step is to attach the pouch, using either an adhesive or mechanical coupling, as described in Chapter 3.

> Some people turn an empty prescription pill bottle upside down, with the top off, and use that to press down on the baseplate around the stoma, ensuring a good seal. Make sure it's the right size bottle. You don't want to press directly on the stoma, just around it.

Many people who have trouble with adherence lie down for 5-10 minutes after putting the baseplate on. Some apply a warm heating pad or lay their warm hand over the appliance during this time, to make sure the adhesive "takes."

## Disposal

Dispose of used baseplates and pouches (and bag liners, if you don't flush them) the same way you'd dispose of soiled diapers.

Avoid plastic grocery bags or anything that isn't air-tight and made to fight odors.

Some people use a diaper disposal system like DIAPER GENIE®. Others don't use the actual apparatus but just the bags that are made for it, which come in a roll. Still others use sealable plastic bags or doggy poop bags. Some brands of ostomy pouches even come with their own odor control trash bags.

Personally, I put my used baseplates, bag liners, and pouches into resealable plastic bags, like freezer bags. Once sealed, they go in a special odor control bag that comes with my pouches. When a few plastic bags have accumulated in there, I tie a knot and throw it out with the regular trash.

# Irrigation

This is only an option for people with descending or sigmoid end colostomies (because your stool needs to be pretty firm, and if you have an ileostomy, irrigating can lead to dehydration). It's basically a water enema, flushing stool out of your colon through the stoma. After you've irrigated, you shouldn't produce any more output for a day or longer, eliminating the need to empty pouches more frequently and irregularly.

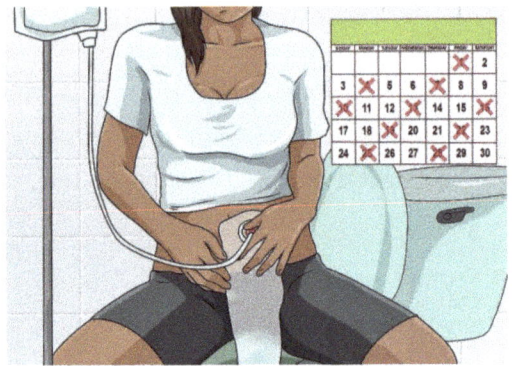

### How it works

You sit on or near a toilet, hang a bag of warm water about shoulder height, like an IV drip, and let the water flow down into your stoma, where it washes out the stool.

The equipment needed is available from ostomy supply companies – basically an irrigation bag (to hold the warm water) with a tube and an on/off flow control valve, a "stoma cone" on the end of the tube that's inserted partway into your stoma (remember that the stoma has no nerve endings, so inserting the cone is painless), and an "irrigation sleeve" that the output flows through and out into the toilet. There are other accessories you might want to use, like an ostomy belt to keep the irrigation sleeve firmly attached to your baseplate, a hook to hang the bag from, and a clip for the end of the sleeve. All easily available.

There's a learning curve at first, of course. You should be taught how to do it by a stoma nurse. There are things to learn, like water temperature, flow rate, how to deal with the odd problem that might crop up, etc.,  but once you've mastered the technique, you may find this a much more attractive option than emptying a pouch frequently.

The whole process usually takes about 45 minutes to an hour. And you only have to do it every day or two, sometimes even every three days.

Following a regular irrigation routine generally works best. You should irrigate the same number of days apart at roughly the same time of day (like every second morning, for example). That doesn't mean you can never change your schedule. If travel, company, or other demands mean you must skip or delay irrigation that's quite alright. Your bowels may take a few days to re-adjust to the variation or they may readily adapt to a new routine.

## Is it for you?

People who irrigate and love it often report ...

- The best part is the freedom that comes from regaining control over your bowel movements.

- After the colon adjusts to this new process and new routine, it typically "learns" to hold the stool inside until the next irrigation. This means that colostomates who successfully irrigate can avoid middle-of-the-night bathroom runs, and embarrassing situations at work or in social situations.

- They can often wear only a small stoma cap or patch in between irrigations, so no bulky appliance.

- They tend to have reduced gas, odor, and skin irritations.

- Irrigation is generally less expensive than frequently replacing pouches.

# TIME FOR A CHANGE

On the downside …

- It can take some time to learn how to irrigate and for your body to adjust to it (at least several weeks).

- Even the most successful irrigators can sometimes have a bit of output in between irrigation sessions. This is usually minor and often in the form of hard pellets. Until you've been irrigating for several months and are familiar with your body's response to irrigation, it's best to carry a spare pouch when you're away from home.

- The time it takes to irrigate is another factor to consider. It takes a lot longer to irrigate than to empty a pouch, although it's done much less often, so if you add up how much time is spent in the bathroom every week, it might even out.

> Some people actually enjoy the forced break of irrigating. They're happy to spend the time listening to music, playing a game on their laptop, reading, etc. while sitting in the bathroom. Others put a clip on the irrigation sleeve, slip into a robe, and putter around the house for a while.

- If you're a bit squeamish about touching your stoma, you'll probably find this whole idea unappealing.

Before making the decision to irrigate, talk it over with a stoma nurse or doctor who's knowledgeable about the process. There are some conditions that have to be ruled out, or at least carefully considered, before starting – such as a prolapsed stoma or hernia, extensive radiation to the lower bowel, and pre-existing conditions like IBD or chronic diarrhea.

**DECISION MATRIX**

|  | *Irrigation* | *Traditional pouch system* |
|---:|:---:|:---:|
| *Feels more "normal" between changes* | **Yes** ✓ | No |
| *Frequency of changes* | **Less** ✓ | More |
| *Urgency/unexpected accidents* | **Less risk** ✓ | More risk |
| *Gas, odor, skin irritation* | **Less** ✓ | More |
| *Appliance can be bulky* | **No** ✓ | Yes |
| *Cost* | **Less** ✓ | More |
| *Hernia, prolapse, pre-existing condition* | Check with doctor | |
| *Ileostomy* | No | **Yes** ✓ |
| *History of bowel problems* | No | **Yes** ✓ |
| *Learning curve / time to adjust* | More | **Less** ✓ |
| *Time in bathroom per change* | More | **Less** ✓ |
| *Need to stick to a routine/schedule* | More | **Less** ✓ |
| *Squeamish about touching stoma?* | No | **Yes** ✓ |

# Chapter Five

# DAILY LIVING

---

*"There is nothing about a stoma that holds you back. It only means you poop out of your belly instead of your butt. If anything, it's more convenient. It's cleaner and its quicker. Beyond that, we all poop, we just do it differently. We still have sex, we still cook and eat, sleep, work, exercise and even take on the same challenges as everyone else."* - **Louise Hunt, Young Crohns: Adventures with a Chronic Illness**

## Sleeping

Remember that your digestive system is working around the clock, cranking out gas and output while you sleep. If you find that your pouch fills up too much overnight, try not to eat for a few hours before bedtime. It's important to stay hydrated, but avoid beverages that could cause gas (like carbonated drinks) or ones that encourage output (like coffee or grape juice, for some people).

> Always check if your pouch needs to be emptied before you go to bed. This should become part of your nighttime ritual, like brushing your teeth.

At first, as your body adjusts to this new set-up, your pouch may need to be emptied during the night – maybe several times. For many ileostomates, this will become their normal routine. Over time, you may find you awaken naturally to empty your pouch. If you're afraid you'll sleep through and experience a leak or blowout, you could set an alarm to wake you every few hours – at least until your body regulates and you can establish a pattern.

Many people get used to waking up a few times to empty and then falling back to sleep. Others rarely need to do this but become attuned to their pouch and can still awaken if it gets too full.

## DAILY LIVING

If you're not used to stumbling around your home, bleary-eyed, in the middle of the night, you might want to install a night light.

If the pouch is inflated with gas, not output, and this is a regular occurrence, you'd probably do best with a pouch that has a filter. See the *Gas* section of the *What Could Possibly Go Wrong?* chapter for more on this subject. In the meantime, you can always release a little gas ("burping" the pouch) and go back to sleep. Just be careful it's only gas in there. You don't want anything else spewing out!

New ostomates often wonder if their whole appliance could fall off during the night, particularly if they move around. The answer is no, unless something's wrong (like being full-to-bursting). Baseplates are surprisingly adherent. They're designed to stay put, day and night. However, for extra peace of mind, you can always wear a belly band or stretchy tube top around your abdomen, to keep everything snug while you sleep.

Keep in mind, though, that a pouch can become so full that it springs a leak. Or even worse, it can pull right off, spilling its contents all over you and your nice clean bed – not to mention your spouse, and possibly the dog! That's why it's a good idea to empty before going to bed, and during the night, if necessary.

If you're concerned about sleeping positions, that's usually not an issue.

- Sleeping on your back is no problem, of course.

- For side sleepers, on the side of your ostomy, the mattress will probably support the pouch. On the opposite side, you might find it helpful to use a small pillow to support it. A travel neck pillow would work well. Personally, I sleep on either side with no problem, and no support pillows. It's never been a problem.

- You can even sleep on your stomach. Many ostomates do. Some bend the leg on the ostomy side to create a little extra room for the bag.

- Bottom line: However you're comfortable is just fine. There's no harm in lying on your pouch (unless it's so full it's about to burst!).

# DAILY LIVING

## Showering & bathing

As soon as your incisions have healed and you're cleared for showering, you're good to go!

You can shower and bathe with the appliance on or off. Both are perfectly fine. Many people shower with the appliance on until it's "change day," when they and their stomas can enjoy complete freedom in the water. If you're having a "naked" shower, just remember not to aim a hard stream of water directly at your stoma. You're not sand-blasting here.

It's possible your stoma could produce output while you're showering with your appliance off. Some people find that eating a few marshmallows about 10-20 minutes earlier will gently "plug them up" for a brief period. If marshmallows don't work for you, maybe you'll discover another food that has that effect, like peanut butter or bananas.

The only drawback to keeping the appliance on is that the pouch stays wet for a while (some brands more than others). You can towel it off or use a blow dryer on a gentle setting. If you find a damp pouch really annoying, you can always cover the appliance first with plastic kitchen wrap, sealing the edges with waterproof tape. Or use PRESS'N SEAL®, a self-sticking plastic film.

> After a shower or bath, tie a baby bib under your pouch to keep the dampness off your skin as it air dries.

If you wear a 2-piece appliance, you can always do a "half-naked" shower - keeping the baseplate on but removing the pouch. This is a particularly good compromise if you're pretty sure you'll have no output for the next few minutes, but it's not time to change your baseplate yet.

There are various "shower guards" on the market - some like plastic aprons, and others like shower caps for the pouch. I've heard of one ostomate using plastic sandwich bags. She makes a vertical slice on one side to slip her pouch through, and puts it on like a rain sleeve, with the opening at the bottom.

## Dressing

Now that you're up and about, you might be wondering if you'll have to change how you dress. The two most common areas of concern are bulges from the ostomy pouch, and waistbands of pants or skirts interfering with the pouch.

**About bulges** – There are several techniques to camouflage bulges.

- Patterned shirts/blouses or pants/skirts.
- Long, loose fitting tops.
- Layering with jackets, sweaters, or long scarves.
- Ostomy wraps or belly bands, to keep the pouch secure and muffle any sounds. Ostomy wraps have one or two inner pockets to tuck the pouch into; belly bands or maternity bands have no inner pockets.

**About waistband**s – Your stoma might be located above your waistline, below it, or smack dab in the middle of it.

**Stoma above waistline** – Your waistband will probably lie across the pouch, so make sure it doesn't restrict the flow of output into the pouch. Elastic waistbands and fabric with some stretch might be all you need. Some women wear maternity pants. Or you could wear low-rise pants, with the waistband sitting under the pouch, and an untucked, loose fitting top to cover it. You could also opt for a stoma guard. It's designed to protect the stoma from injury, like an athletic cup, but will also protect the pouch from being squashed by the waistband.

**Stoma at waistline** – You don't want the waistband to press against your stoma. A stoma guard would work here too. Or you could wear low-rise pants, with the waistband under or over the pouch. If it's under the pouch, you could wear untucked, loose fitting tops, and if it's over the pouch, elastic waistbands and stretchy fabric might be all you need.

# DAILY LIVING

**Stoma below waistline** – To make sure the waistband doesn't press on your stoma, mid-rise or high-rise pants/skirts are your best bet. If you can't find anything that clears the stoma, a stoma guard is another option.

**Ostomy pouch covers** – If you wear pants or skirts with the waistband under the pouch (so it hangs out), or across it (with the top peeking out), you might be concerned about it being accidentally exposed, even when covered by a long top or layers. You may feel more secure with a fabric cover that fits over your pouch. Many ostomates aren't concerned at all about their pouches showing (on the beach, for example), and consider pouch covers a fashion accessory. Others feel more confident and attractive when they wear covers during intimate moments.

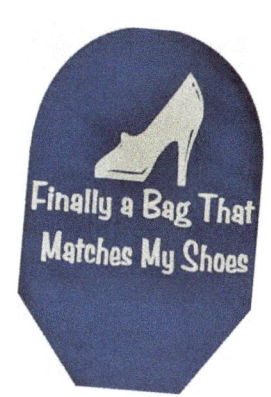

Covers are made to slip easily over a pouch. They're available commercially, and many people make their own. They can be fun and attractive. Whether your style is "manly" camouflage patterns, hippie tie dye, sexy black lace, sassy sayings, or superheros, the only limit is your imagination.

## Eating & drinking

Like everyone else, what we eat and drink has a tremendous effect on our daily lives. Many of the challenges we face can be reduced or even eliminated by diet.

Be particularly careful in the first 6-8 weeks after surgery, when your stoma can be swollen and blockages can happen more easily. During this period, avoid tough stringy meats, foods with skins (even corn or peas), sausage casings, popcorn, coconut, and other foods that are hard to digest.

DAILY LIVING

It's better for your digestive system to process six small meals a day than three big ones. So if you like to "graze," knock yourself out! Now you have a good medical excuse.

Chew foods really well, especially those than can cause blockage, like popcorn, stringy meats, and large pieces of leafy greens. Spit out anything that may cause a problem. In my pre-ostomy days, I often swallowed meat gristle, watermelon seeds, and hard bits of popcorn without a second thought. Nowadays I'm much more selective about what I swallow.

The 11th commandment for ostomates is "Thou shalt stay hydrated!" This table shows some examples of how much water is generally recommended, based on body weight:

| If you weigh: | You should drink (daily): |
|---|---|
| 100 lbs / 50 kilos | 1½ quarts / litres |
| 140 lbs / 65 kilos | 2 quarts / litres |
| 180 lbs / 80 kilos | 3 quarts / litres |
| 220 lbs / 100 kilos | 3½ quarts / litres |

Don't be intimidated. The amount I should drink seems high to me too and frankly I consider it more of a target, but I try. Remember this means water from all sources. You also get water from food, like fruits and vegetables, and from all sorts of beverages. Just keep in mind that a cup of coffee or a glass of soda isn't equivalent to exactly that much water. You get more bang for your buck with water, and a little less with other drinks.

People react differently to different foods. Something that may be well tolerated by one person can trigger problems in another. If you're unsure about trying certain foods, keep a food diary. Make a note of what you eat every day and how your digestive system is working – basically, what goes in and what comes out.

You might see patterns you weren't aware of, learning what foods you can enjoy and which ones you should avoid.

Add new foods one at a time, waiting a couple of days to see if they agree with you before adding another new one.

### Some special notes for ileostomates:

Your food is processed only in the small intestine before exiting your body. It bypasses the large intestine – where cellulose (fiber) is digested. So in ileostomates, fiber generally passes out of the body undigested. But sometimes it can collect in there, causing a blockage. Small quantities of fiber shouldn't be a problem, but particularly in the first 6-8 weeks after surgery, be very careful.

After that, you can help break down the cellulose yourself by cooking foods that are higher in fiber, chopping them into small pieces, and chewing them well. Some people call this the "3 C's" – cook, chop, and chew. Try to chew until your food is the consistency of baby food.

Many ileostomates find it simpler to follow a low-fiber diet, to reduce the risk of complications like food blockages. See the *Food Tables* (Appendix A) for recommendations.

### Nutrients & vitamins

Because nutrients from the food you eat are absorbed as they pass through your digestive system, it's important to know at what point they're being diverted out through your stoma. Many ostomates don't have this information. If you don't know, ask your doctor.

Here are some examples of why it matters:

- Some people with ileostomies or "short bowel syndrome" may not get enough Vitamin B12 from their food, because it's absorbed in the part of the small intestine their food doesn't reach – mostly in the bottom part of the small intestine, called the ileum. A B12 deficiency can lead to several

# DAILY LIVING

symptoms, including constipation/diarrhea, memory loss, and feelings of being weak, tired, or depressed. If you have a deficiency in this important vitamin you should take a supplement in liquid form, by injection, or by nasal spray. If taken in pill form, it may not be fully absorbed before it passes out through your stoma (see the *Medications* section, below).

- Much of the electrolytes (including sodium and potassium) that your body needs are absorbed in the large intestine. If your stoma is located before the large intestine (as in ileostomies), or if you've lost a lot of your colon (like a colostomy closer to the beginning of the large intestine), you might need more electrolytes in your diet.

- Vitamin K, which plays a big role in blood clotting, is produced and absorbed in the large intestine. If you're having trouble with bruising or excessive bleeding, ask your doctor if this could be the reason. A supplement might be recommended.

Many more nutrients and vitamins are absorbed along the way. The more intestines are bypassed by your ostomy, the more important it is to consult with a registered dietician or nutritionist to find out what foods or supplements you should be taking, to replace what you're not getting naturally.

## Medications

You may take several medications, for medical reasons and/or to replace nutrients, vitamins, and minerals. It's important to make sure that the pills are completely absorbed. Basically, the closer your stoma is located to your rectum (or where your rectum used to be), the less you need to worry about this. It's a particular problem for ileostomates, who

> Unsure if your pills are being absorbed properly? Drop one in a glass of water. If it hasn't started to dissolve in half an hour, you should try the medication in another format.

# DAILY LIVING

may find that pills pass through their stomas looking very much like they did when they went in – because they haven't had a chance to be absorbed.

For ileostomates, medication is generally best taken in liquid form, by injection, or by nasal sprays. Some, but not all, ileostomates find that gel capsules, quick dissolving or uncoated tablets work for them. But avoid pills that are coated (called an enteric coating) to make it easier on the stomach, or those designed for slow release (extended or sustained release products).

If it's an uncoated pill or tablet, you could crush it and mix it in with a spoonful of jam or water. But don't try this with time release tablets or gel caps without checking with your doctor or pharmacist first.

## Getting organized

Ostomies come with a lot of baggage that can clutter up your home and your mind. Try to get a handle on all that clutter before it engulfs you.

Within a few weeks of surgery, you'll be awash in ostomy supplies and paraphernalia. The place where you change your appliance can start to look like a M.A.S.H. unit. That's not good for you psychologically, and not very pleasant for family members or visitors either. You'll all feel more positive if you can get it back to looking more homey, and less like a hospital.

> Donate unused supplies to one of the many organizations that distribute ostomy products to people in need, locally or in developing countries. You'll feel good to be helping others, while enjoying all that freed-up space.

Try to have all your supplies within easy reach when needed, but out of sight the rest of the time.

# DAILY LIVING

Everyone's needs and available space are different but to use my own situation as an example, here's what worked best in my tiny bathroom:

- A plastic container set of 3 drawers on wheels, tucked away behind the door, within reach of the toilet. Inexpensive but very effective.

    - In the top two drawers, I keep my stash of supplies - baseplates, pouches, bag liners, resealable plastic bags, and odor control bags.

    - The bottom drawer is for leftovers - sample products I may try sometime, and products I don't need every day but want to have ready in case of skin irritations, etc. I also keep my well-bagged used baseplates, pouches, and a box of bag liners in there, awaiting disposal. "Leftovers" in the true sense of the word! When I remember, I toss in a scented dryer sheet, just to be extra sure things stay fresh.

- On top of the toilet tank is a mirror (positioned so I can see what I'm doing when facing the toilet), and a small acrylic chest of 3 more drawers. I don't know what it was meant for. Maybe jewelry or makeup? It's attractive, and the perfect size for small ostomy products - like packets of adhesive remover, barrier rings, ostomy scissors, and about a week's worth of bag liners.

- The result is that I can stand in front of the toilet, see what I'm doing, and reach everything I need without taking a step. But when I'm not changing my appliance, everything's tucked away behind closed drawers and no-one would ever guess my bathroom is "ostomy central."

Taking care of an ostomy is very hands-on. But a little paperwork can be helpful too - like a food journal, where you keep track of new foods you try and note if they had any effect.

It's also handy to have a notebook to record medical information. This can be as simple as the names and contact information of your doctors, stoma nurse, and whoever you order supplies from, the product numbers of your ostomy supplies, a list of your current medications, the date(s) of your operation(s), and the type of surgery you had, including what part of your intestines were affected. Bring this with you to medical appointments or ER visits so you can answer questions without looking like a deer in the headlights. You'd be surprised how easy it is to forget details, particularly if you're under stress.

Bottom line: Show your ostomy who's boss. As much as you can, take control of your environment and the management of your ostomy. This will leave you time to get back to more important things, like enjoying the rest of your life.

## Finding support

New ostomates can feel they're alone in the world. Most of us never knew anyone who had one. In addition to feeling lonely, you may also experience emotions like anger or depression, and be overwhelmed with questions about living with this strange new object on your stomach.

The best solution to all these concerns is to talk to others. Of course, you should turn to doctors and nurses for medical advice. But people who are actually living with ostomies are a great source of information and support in a whole range of other areas. So how do you find them? Here are two good ways:

### Online groups

There are many online groups to choose from. Some specialize in things like ostomies in children, or in people with other complex medical issues. Others are simply for anyone with an ostomy, and their caregivers. They're easy to find by searching terms like "ostomy support group online." Typically, all you need to do is sign up with an email address.

Many of these groups are private. That means only other members can post messages and respond to others. Some are semi-private. Anyone can read the posts but you have to be a member to post a message or respond.

Most (if not all) groups are moderated. That means someone's in charge, to remind members of rules, like whether or not photos of stomas are allowed and if so, where and how to post them. Moderators generally read all posts, delete anything inappropriate, and can even block offending members. The job of a good moderator is to keep everyone feeling safe and comfortable.

You might want to try a few groups on for size, to find one that feels most natural for you.

Don't be afraid to share or ask anything, even if it seems embarrassing or trivial. There's nothing you can say that will shock anyone. If you stepped in poo on the way to the bathroom, these are the folks who can relate and laugh about it with you. If you're overwhelmed and feel you can't cope one minute longer, these are the folks who will embrace you with virtual hugs, and let you know you're not alone. And if you're wondering what to expect from an upcoming medical procedure, who better to ask than people who've "been there, done that"?

When you post a message about an issue you're having, always start off by saying what type of ostomy you have – urostomy, ileostomy or colostomy. Remember that the people answering you aren't doctors. They're well-meaning and often very knowledgeable, but some might unknowingly give you advice that works for them and their type of ostomy, but isn't right for you.

Overall, online ostomy groups are an incredibly rich source of information and support. It's like joining a private club with members all over the world. Only instead of a secret handshake, we recognize each other in public from the stealthy 'ostomy pat-down' signal – a discreet patting of the small bulge on our tummies, to check for inflation. We're out there, in the thousands, ready to offer a helping hand or just listen to a fellow club member. So join up and take full advantage of this wonderful resource.

**ETIQUETTE TIPS FOR ONLINE SUPPORT GROUPS**

**Lurk for a while.** You don't have to start posting right away. Spend some time reading the posts of others. This will give you a feel for the tone of the group, and if it's a place you think you'd be comfortable.

**Introduce yourself.** When you're ready, share a little background on why you have an ostomy, what type you have, and any current issues you're dealing with.

**Respond to others' posts.** You aren't expected to be a medical expert. Even if you don't have an answer to a problem, people still appreciate a word of encouragement. Obviously, you don't need to respond to every single post. But if you have anything helpful or supportive to say, don't hesitate.

**Share what works for you**, and what doesn't. Everyone's different, but if something helped you, it will probably help someone else. It doesn't have to be medical. For example, you might get comfort or strength from meditation, yoga, medical marijuana, or prayer. That's always nice to share. Just, please, don't insist that people who don't think the same way you do are wrong. Everyone should feel safe and accepted.

**Welcome others.** Someone new to the wonderful world of ostomies might feel timid about asking what seems like an obvious question. Sure, it's probably been asked a thousand times before, but it's all new to *this* person. If you can, take a few minutes to answer the question and make them feel welcomed.

DAILY LIVING

## Local groups

If you prefer face-to-face meetings, those are pretty widely available too. Most cities have at least one ostomy support group.

Ask your doctor or stoma nurse if they know of one. If there's an ostomy society in your area, they should certainly know. You could also ask associations for conditions that frequently lead to ostomies, like cancer, or an inflammatory bowel disease.

If there isn't a group near you and if you're up to it, you might consider starting one yourself. You just need a few people to start with, and a place to meet.

Again, your doctor or stoma nurse might be of help here. Write up a little blurb about wanting to start a group and ask them to give it to any patients who might be interested. Or post a flyer on a bulletin board at your hospital. If you're a member of an online group, ask if there are other members in your area who'd be interested in forming a local group.

In the beginning, you could meet in someone's home, maybe taking turns. Community centers, hospitals, and churches will often make meeting rooms available for groups like this. You don't need much. A few chairs. Maybe a coffee machine.

Once it gets going, you might want to invite a guest speaker from time to time. Like a colorectal surgeon, or gastroenterologist, or stoma nurse.

Whether online or in person, connecting with other ostomates can make a huge difference in your life. There are a few million people with ostomies in the world, and thousands more each year. There's no need to feel alone. They're out there, wanting to talk to someone too.

# Chapter Six

## OUT & ABOUT

---

*"When you're a person with a chronic illness and have a medical device that you can't live without, there are always going to be things that don't function quite right. However, that should never stop you from going out and enjoying life the way you want to live it."* - **Jessica Grossman, uncoverostomy.org**

Okay, so you've been home from the hospital for a while, you've gotten more or less comfortable with changing your appliance, you've established a daily routine, and you're finally ready to venture out. Congratulations! Your "new normal" life awaits. And the more prepared you are, the easier it will be.

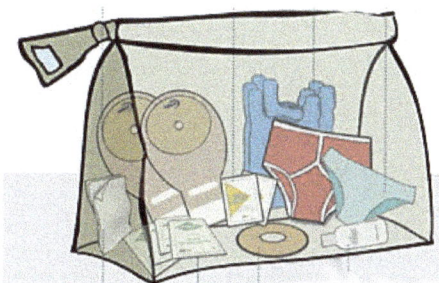

## Emergency kit

Ostomates learn to expect the unexpected. Never go too far from home, or for too long, without back-up supplies. A toiletry or makeup bag packed with everything you'll need for a complete appliance change can be a lifesaver.

## OUT & ABOUT

Here are some typical products to include:

> **Baseplate & pouch** – ideally, with a pre-cut hole.
>
> **Ostomy scissors/template** – if you haven't pre-cut the hole but will need to.
>
> **Gauze or some type of soft wipes** – for cleaning the skin. Baby wipes are good to have, in case there's no access to water.
>
> **Products you routinely use** – like bag liners, lubricating oil, stoma powder, barrier spray or wipes, moldable rings, paste, adhesive remover, etc.
>
> **Trash bag/resealable plastic bag** – for easy disposal of used products.
>
> **Folding mirror** – to put on a toilet tank or shelf, so you can see what you're doing ... if you're lucky enough to be in a public bathroom that has such things!
>
> **Hand sanitizer** – you may not be near a sink.
>
> **Deodorizer**, if you're concerned about odors – to spritz the air, or spray on the toilet water.

Of course, how many supplies you pack depends on your own needs and how long you'll be gone. This is particularly true of baseplates and pouches. I always keep at least two of each in my kit. Not only for when I'm out, but also as a back-up in case my regular supply runs out at home. It's kind of like tucking away a little cash in a drawer for emergencies. Out of sight, out of mind – until you're unexpectedly caught short one day, then you're so grateful for that secret stash!

# OUT & ABOUT

Some suppliers provide canvas bags to use as emergency kits. I've received a few from stoma nurses. Or you could call suppliers directly and ask if they offer them as free gifts to customers. These bags typically hold enough for a few complete changes.

If you need even more space for your supplies, several ostomates find diaper bags are the perfect size. They're usually filled with partitions and pockets to keep things organized. Some are made of leather, and look like any roomy, good quality, over the shoulder bag.

> Be sure to replenish supplies in your kit as soon as you get home, and keep it somewhere handy so you can grab it at a moment's notice.

It's also handy to leave an emergency kit in places you frequent – like your car or office, or school locker. One caveat: excessive heat can damage the adhesive on baseplates. So if you're in a hot climate, leaving the kit in your glove compartment or trunk for prolonged periods isn't the best plan.

You don't want them to freeze in cold weather either. If you don't have time to warm up the baseplate, it may not adhere properly.

Women can easily toss an emergency kit into a roomy purse or tote bag, but men need to be a little more creative. I've heard of men using coat pockets, backpacks, fanny packs, briefcases, laptop bags, and cross-body or messenger bags. And of course, like women, they can always leave a stash of supplies in the car.

Some people also keep a roll of paper towels or a change of clothes in the car or at work, in case of a blowout or significant leak.

Interestingly, I've heard many more men than women say they never take extra supplies when they go out and have never had a problem. I guess that's the ostomy equivalent of 'going commando.' Of course, it's also the ostomy equivalent of Russian roulette!

OUT & ABOUT

## Hospital stays

If you have to go to an ER or be admitted for any reason, try to bring your own supplies. Don't expect that they'll have a stock of ostomy products on hand – let alone the specific brands and types you're currently using.

If you're having a procedure directly related to your ostomy, you can assume the medical team will know what they're doing. But others may be totally unfamiliar with the needs of an ostomate or how to change an appliance. You may have to teach *them!*

If you're an ileostomate experiencing a blockage, take the UOAA's *Ileostomy Blockage Guide* (Appendix C) with you.

This is a good time to wear a 2-piece appliance or bag liners, even if you normally don't. It's much easier to simply remove the pouch or liner, dispose of it, and replace it, than to change a baseplate or go through the whole emptying process – particularly if your mobility is temporarily reduced. If you've brought your own odor-control trash bags, you may not even need to get out of bed!

## Public bathrooms

Changing an appliance or even just emptying a pouch in a public bathroom can be a challenge, to say the least. Stalls are cramped, there's usually nowhere to prop up a mirror or lay out supplies, and toilets are often very low. If you have no option, do the best you can, even if it's a "quick & dirty" job. Then check it out as soon as you get home. You may need to do a more thorough cleaning or change the appliance entirely.

Using a handicapped bathroom is much easier. These facilities often include a shelf, and sometimes even a sink. The toilets can be higher, so easier to get on and off for someone who's had stomach surgery. There's usually a bar to grab onto for that reason too. Plus just having more space and privacy is a huge relief.

In Japan, some public bathrooms post an icon showing that they have facilities for people with ostomies. But in most of our uncivilized world, this is a fantasy. In fact, you might get an occasional glare or unpleasant remark when you emerge from a handicapped stall in a public bathroom, because you appear able-bodied. How to handle that is of course up to you, but it may help to have a response ready. Some people explain they have an ostomy, or an invisible handicap. Some feel they don't owe an explanation to anybody. And others seize the opportunity to jump on their soapboxes and loudly proclaim their rights. Your call.

My daughter (a non-ostomate) is wheelchair-bound. She's often had to suffer in pain to reach a handicapped bathroom, only to find it occupied by a seemingly able-bodied person who just wanted more room to put down shopping bags or try on new clothes. But my daughter knows there are people like me too, without a visible handicap, who actually need the facilities. So she doesn't jump to conclusions. A little tolerance on both sides goes a long way.

If you spring a leak, you need to move swiftly. I like to scout out public places where I go frequently, and locate the best bathrooms. For instance, in my hospital there are several bathrooms with a handicapped stall, but also a couple of stand-alone, unisex, full bathrooms, complete with a sink. Almost as good as home! I keep a treasure map in my head, showing the locations of these hidden gems.

## Back to work

Returning to work with an ostomy presents a few unique challenges. Here are some tips that can help make it easier.

> **Check with your doctor** – Get a medical all-clear from your doctor or stoma nurse. How soon you can return to work depends very much on the kind of work you do. If it involves heavy lifting, for example, you may need to wait longer or actually change your duties. It might be recommended that you return gradually – maybe fewer hours or days per week at first. Or perhaps you could tele-commute for a while.

**Advance planning** - Take the time to carefully consider how your ostomy might affect you at work. Think about everything, from uniforms to toilet facilities. This way you can problem-solve in advance and be prepared with practical solutions.

**To tell or not to tell?** - Whoever you report to should be aware you have an ostomy. Explain what impact, if any, this might have on your day-to-day work and offer your solutions to situations that might arise. For example, if you're an air traffic controller or a server in a restaurant, you can't just suddenly nip off to empty your pouch without calling in a temporary replacement. Those arrangements and any others specific to your particular job need to be worked out with your employer before you return. So you should tell at least that one person. What, if anything, you choose to tell any other co-workers about your ostomy is entirely up to you and your comfort level.

**Be prepared** - Keep a fully-stocked emergency kit at your workplace. Personally, I'd keep at least a week's worth of supplies on hand, including several resealable plastic bags and odor control bags, so I wouldn't have to replenish the kit daily or risk being caught short. Many folks leave a change of clothes at work too, for peace of mind.

**Using the facilities** - Your workplace might have a stand-alone bathroom, like at home, or a communal one with cubicles. If you'll require a private sink occasionally or even with every change, and the facilities are communal, you may need to make other arrangements. Perhaps there's a private bathroom for higher-ups that you could seek permission to use.

One of your primary concerns will probably be about smells. See the *Smells* section of Chapter 7 for tips on how to reduce odors in your bag, in the toilet, and in the air.

Leaving used pouches or appliances in a trash receptacle in a common area, even if they're well bagged, is probably not the best plan. Instead, seal them well (e.g., in a resealable plastic bag, inside an odor control bag) and keep them in your personal space, like in a drawer or locker, until you can take them home and dispose of them there.

If you feel awkward carrying a little trash bag and emergency kit in and out of the bathroom, you could always keep them in an attractive shoe bag or leather satchel of some kind. That way, you could stop and chat with co-workers en route without feeling uncomfortable. You might even develop an aura of mystique. For all they know, there are closely guarded national secrets in there, or a flask of gin. LOL. If they only knew!

**Noises** – Everyone "breaks wind" sometimes. The only difference is whether the sound comes from behind or in front of them. Either way, it can be embarrassing, particularly in a work situation.

It can help to avoid foods that produce gas (see *Food Tables*, Appendix A), and you can wear an ostomy band or belly wrap, or even a stoma guard, to help muffle the sounds. But you can never guarantee that your stoma won't suddenly speak up in public.

> Lisa Goodman-Helfand, a gifted author and professional speaker on healthcare issues (www.comfortableinmythickskin.com), admits that her stoma *"... can produce flatulent noises that are very difficult to ignore for even the most polite adult. Other times, my stoma generates loud gurgling noises akin to a drain that's just been unclogged. When these embarrassing sounds escape, I have a menu of canned responses I can select from:*
>
> **Option #1 (tell a lie):** "Oh, excuse me, my stomach is growling, I forgot to eat breakfast this morning." This is typically met with a weak smile that's betraying the person's body language which reads: Uh-huh, sure.
>
> **Option #2 (tell the truth):** "Sorry, my stomach makes weird noises because I don't have a colon. The good news is, I'm not really farting, so no need to anticipate a foul odor." I only say this to people who already know about my surgery, as it would be an odd thing to say to a stranger or acquaintance and I already feel like I come off weird enough.

**Option #3**: Ignore the fact that I'm a human fart noise machine and just pretend I didn't notice."

Sometimes you can crack a joke to break an awkward silence. For example, if your stoma makes that unmistakable sound in front of co-workers who know you're an ostomate, you could dart a glance at your tummy and stage-whisper "Hush up. No-one cares what you think!" Yes, it's embarrassing. But that ship has sailed. The best you can do now is show others it's no big deal. They'll probably be relieved, share a chuckle, and get back to what they were talking about.

# Travel

Travelling with an ostomy can be easy-peazy. It just takes a little thinking ahead.

## General travel tips

If you'll be away from home for an extended period, check if there's a local source to buy ostomy supplies. Even if you're sure you've packed enough, you'll feel more secure knowing back-ups are available.

Try to keep to your usual eating practices while you're away. This is no time to try something new and exotic, or to treat yourself to something you know will make you gassy or affect your output in a significant way.

> Anticipate how many supplies you'll need for the days you'll be away ... then <u>double or triple it</u>. Nothing's worse than being stranded without supplies when you're away from home.

If you feel the local water might be a little iffy, use bottled water – not just for drinking, but also for washing your stoma area and rinsing out your pouches. If you thought travelers' diarrhea was bad before, imagine having it with an ostomy!

## Hotels

Staying at a hotel is nothing to worry about. It just takes a little consideration. The most common concern is what to do about the disposal of used ostomy supplies. Resealable plastic bags and odor control bags (preferably not transparent) are the solution here. They can be deposited in a bathroom trash basket, which is emptied daily.

Chambermaids have said that compared to some of the indescribable messes they've had to clean up (visions of rock stars with goats in their rooms and body fluids dripping down the walls), a well-sealed, non-smelling, tidily packaged bag of poop isn't worth a second thought. If the outside bag isn't see-through, they'll probably never realize what's in it anyway. And even if they did, they'd appreciate the trouble you took.

Another concern about hotel stays is the potential of soiling bed sheets. For peace of mind, you can always pack a few disposable incontinence pads to sleep on, laid over the bottom sheet. If a pad gets soiled, it can be placed in a plastic bag too. So bring some larger odor control trash bags if you think there's a risk, and double bag if necessary.

In the worst-case scenario, if a bit of a mess happens, don't panic. Just call the housekeeping department and explain your situation. Again, they've seen things a thousand times worse. This is their job. And if you happen to run into an employee who resents it, then blow it off. It means they have a much bigger problem than your little accident.

## Being a houseguest

Staying at someone's home raises many of the same concerns as staying at a hotel, or on a cruise ship for that matter.

Resealable plastic bags and odor control bags can solve any disposal problems. But rather than leaving the bags in a waste basket in the bathroom, particularly one that's shared with others, you could always keep the bags in your own bedroom until they can be deposited in an outdoor garbage can.

For extra peace of mind, you can pack a bottle of a nice-smelling essential oil and some cotton balls. Dab a few drops of oil on a cotton ball and put it wherever you're keeping your "bag of bags." Freshen as needed.

If you're staying in someone's home, it's probably a friend or family member who knows about your ostomy. So you should feel comfortable asking where you can dispose of your sealed bags. Maybe there's a garbage can in the garage. When do they put out the trash for pick-up? When they realize this is no big deal for you, just a minor detail that's easy to accommodate, they'll feel more relaxed about it too.

Actually, if this is your first visit since having an ostomy, your hosts may have their own questions they're hesitant to ask. Like most of us before our surgeries, they're probably totally clueless about how this ostomy business works. So if you're comfortable, bring it up in conversation prior to your visit. Let them know if there's anything they can do to ensure a relaxed and happy experience for everyone.

For example, if you have any dietary issues – like doing best with a low residue or high fiber diet, or needing to avoid particular foods because they've caused you blockages in the past – give your hosts a heads-up. There's nothing more frustrating than laying out a lovely spread for guests, only to suddenly learn that Uncle Joe's new wife is deathly allergic to shellfish and cousin Shlomo just turned vegan! In the same way, they won't want to feed you anything that will cause you discomfort. So give them a chance to do a little menu planning before your visit. They'll appreciate it.

## Air travel

A lot of people flying with an ostomy for the first time are apprehensive about airport security checks. Although many airport personnel have been taught about ostomies, you can't always rely on that. You might prefer to tell them you have an ostomy before they start eyeing that suspicious bulge under your shirt.

## OUT & ABOUT

You can carry a doctor's note explaining that you have an ostomy, or print out a "Travel Communication Card" created for that purpose by the United Ostomy Associations of America, Inc. (available on their website). This doesn't guarantee you won't be screened or patted down, but it can come in handy if you're dealing with a security officer who just doesn't get it.

They might ask you to rub your hand over your pouch (on the outside of your clothing), and then test your hand to make sure there's no residue of an explosive. That's pretty standard and nothing to worry about.

Keep your supplies with you. This is definitely carry-on material, not checked baggage. You don't want to land in Cabo San Lucas, only to find that your ostomy supplies are winging their way to France! Besides, even if you eventually got them back, they'd probably be very snooty and burp with a French accent.

If you cut your own baseplate holes, cut them all before you leave. You could pack ostomy scissors in your travel kit, but rules on the size of scissors you're allowed to carry on a plane can vary by jurisdiction. In some countries, you can't bring any scissors onto the aircraft with you. Again, this is a better safe than sorry scenario. If you must carry scissors, it's best to put them in your checked luggage.

Check out the rules for liquids too. Your bottles of lubricating oil or hand sanitizer might exceed the limits on size or quantity. At many airports, medical supplies are ok if they're labelled and prescribed. But you never know when you'll run into a customs or security agent who got up on the wrong side of the bed that morning and wants to be difficult. The odds are probably in your favor but personally, I'd rather do my gambling in Vegas.

Be especially careful about eating or drinking before a flight, and empty your pouch shortly before boarding, to reduce the need to burp or empty it en route. Also, don't consume anything during the flight that you know from experience might cause gas or excessive output. Airplane bathrooms are hardly big enough to change your mind, let alone an ostomy pouch!

# OUT & ABOUT

Many ostomates have heard that air pressure can cause the gas inside an ostomy pouch to expand slightly at high altitudes. There have been some scientific studies to suggest this, in theory. But I've never heard of it actually happening in real life – at least not to the extent of the pouch being pulled off someone's abdomen or "exploding" (as some people fear). In fact, there are many other reasons why you may experience a little more gas on an airplane, causing the pouch to balloon slightly. But as long as you have a filter that works, and burp your pouch if necessary, you'll be just fine.

## Road trips or camping

The main challenge here, of course, is limited access to toilet facilities. Or even none at all. But don't let that put you off. You just have to be more creative.

A good trick is to have something you can line with a plastic bag. Could be a coffee can, a big glass jar, or a plastic food container – anything with a tight-fitting lid. Line it with a plastic bag, empty your ostomy pouch or drop your used appliance into it, and cover it with the lid until you can tie up the plastic bag and dispose of it.

Obviously, you're going to need a well-stocked kit of supplies, including packets of wipes and hand sanitizers, and lots of plastic bags.

Keep bottled water on hand to help with cleaning & rinsing.

At least one company makes a nifty device that's essentially a folding plastic bucket you strap around your waist. Again, you line it with a plastic bag, empty your output (and anything else, like used wipes, used baseplates, etc.) into the bucket, tie up the bag, and dispose of it. The main advantages here are that you can do a complete change with both hands, while standing or sitting, and you don't have to worry about your stoma leaking while it's exposed. Everything will fall into the bag-lined bucket. It's a great solution to the problem of pouch changes when there are no bathrooms around.

Used plastic bags can be disposed of in various ways. If you've emptied only output into a biodegradable bag (i.e., no foil-wrapped wipes or other non-biodegradables), you can bury it in the woods. Otherwise, hang onto the tied-up bags until you can put them in a trash receptacle. You should have a supply of larger odor-controlled bags to collect them in, until the right opportunity arises.

# Swimming

Many new ostomates wonder if they'll be able to swim again.

### Can you do it?

Absolutely! By far, most people with ostomies report that they can swim freely in pools and oceans, for any length of time, and in any temperature of water, with no problems. Many are scuba diving, surfing, and waterskiing like they used to.

Of course, like any other aspect of life with an ostomy, there are individual differences. A few people have reported that their baseplate loosens after prolonged exposure to water, or in a hot tub, or that salt water affects the baseplate's adhesion. They're a really small minority, but you won't know for sure how it will be for you until you try. So take a deep breath, hold your nose, and jump in!

If your pouch has a filter (allowing gas to escape), cover it with a sticker that probably came with your pouches. An uncovered filter won't work if it gets wet or clogged with sand.

After the swim, you might find the baseplate is harder than usual to remove. That's because some of them are made to grip on even tighter when wet - which is reassuring, actually. Just remember that you might need to let it dry out before peeling it off.

## What about leaking?

It's natural to worry about leaking while swimming. If you're not normally prone to leaking on dry land, it's not likely to be any different in the water. But here are some tips that can boost your sense of security.

You can refrain from eating or drinking in the hours before swimming, particularly if you know you have a short transit time (how long it takes food to travel through your system).

Some people find that eating specific foods, like marshmallows or peanut butter, holds off output for a while. That doesn't work for everyone, but you might find a food that works for you.

Don't swim immediately after applying a new baseplate. Let some time pass to allow the adhesive to bond to your skin and ensure a really secure seal. At least 15 minutes. A few hours would be even better.

Many swimmers use waterproof tape to make sure their appliances are extra secure from leaking or loosening. Two particular favorites are MEDIPORE® and HY-TAPE® (AKA "pink tape"), applied like a picture frame around the baseplate.

Flange extenders can also provide added security. They're not specifically made for swimming, but to protect against leakage or loosening generally, and they can go in water like any ostomy product. These are typically C-shaped or Y-shaped "peel and stick" strips that go around the edge of the baseplate.

A lot of people use a self-sticking plastic film like PRESS'N SEAL® to prevent leaks coming out or water coming in while swimming. Lay a big square across your stomach, completely covering your appliance and surrounding skin. Then press it firmly all over so it sticks to the appliance and to your stomach. It should remain in place throughout your swim.

You can use any of these products (waterproof tape, flange extenders, and self-sticking plastic film) alone or in combination with each other.

If you're still nervous about your first post-ostomy swim, why not do a test run in a bath? Sit in the tub with your appliance submerged for about a half hour, then check for any leaks or loosening around the edges of the baseplate. If there's a problem, you can use some of the tips above. If all's well, any lingering doubts should disappear down the drain along with the bath water.

### What should you wear?

As ostomy awareness grows, more and more ostomates are comfortable exposing their appliances, with or without attractive covers. Others are more comfortable knowing they're fully covered.

> Whether you're the "I'm here, I've got gear, get used to it!" type or someone who wants total disguise and coverage, there's a swimsuit out there with your name on it.

There are bathing suits and swim wraps specially designed for ostomates, many with front panels to reduce the profile of your appliance, or inner pockets to tuck the pouch into. However, most swimmers don't find these necessary.

Women have lots of choices in swimwear. If your ostomy is low enough, you can wear a regular two-piece suit. If it's higher, there are two-piece suits with high waisted bottoms. Tankinis are another great option. Many of the tops are long and flowy, disguising any bulges. One-piece suits are popular too, and back in style. Skirts and ruching can help to disguise any bumps or bulges from your appliance, and suits with control panels will help keep the pouch snug against your tummy.

## OUT & ABOUT

Men can wear boxer-type swim trunks or swim shorts – as opposed to tight fitting briefs – although some wear briefs under the roomier trunks, to keep the pouch snug.

On the beach or poolside, sarongs and wraps are perfect for women with & without ostomies, and long, roomy T-shirts are great cover-ups for both sexes.

If you're still concerned about your appliance creating a bulge, there are small pouches called stoma caps, designed to hold only a tiny bit of output. They're good for short periods like swimming, when you may want your appliance to be as unobtrusive as possible. Just be sure you can count on your stoma to behave itself.

If you're wearing a full-size pouch and are concerned that it might peek out from the bottom of your swimsuit, you can always put it on sideways, with the pouch laying horizontally across your stomach.

Alternatively, you can fold it up from the bottom, so it's doubled over your stoma. The bathing suit might hold it in place, but you could also use the PRESS'N SEAL® plastic film tip here, to keep it securely folded.

If you wear a hernia belt, there's no reason you can't wear it under your bathing suit. Just remember to have a dry one ready to put on when you change back into your clothes, and to hand wash the wet one before wearing it again, to get rid of any chlorine, salt, sand, etc.

# Chapter Seven
# WHAT COULD POSSIBLY GO WRONG?

*The way we deal with the crazy situations in which only ostomates find ourselves varies person to person, and that doesn't mean any one response is better than another. And there are some times where all the preparation in the world can't save you from a Poopmageddon. So in those unexpected, undocumented, unfortunate moments, I have learned to take a minute to recognize all of those emotions, take a deep breath, and handle the situation."* – **Molly Atwater, @MollyOllyOstomy**

What could go wrong? Well, um, a number of things, actually – from the benign and inconvenient to the more serious. The only thing you can count on is that something probably *will* happen sooner or later. It's part of the package. But take heart. There are loads of ideas and products out there to help you.

## Smells

"Is it me or the dog?" Worrying about smells is a common preoccupation for ostomates.

First, remember that it may not be as bad as you think. Ostomates are often convinced there's an odor coming from their pouch, even when friends and loved ones insist there's nothing. We tend to be overly sensitive about it.

A properly sealed pouch shouldn't emit any odors at all, so if you're sure there's a smell coming from it, check for leaks.

If your pouch has a filter (designed to let gas out but keep odors in), it could mean that the filter is clogged.

# WHAT COULD POSSIBLY GO WRONG?

If you want an extra boost of confidence, sprinkle a drop of two of an essential oil on the outside of your pouch. I use an orange oil, but there are lots of choices. It helps you feel fresh & clean.

It's true that some people's poop smells more than others', and can vary with different foods. See the *Eating & Drinking* section for more on that. And it's generally believed that the output from a colostomy is stronger smelling than that of an ileostomy, because it consists of fully formed stool.

## In the pouch

There are a few things you could try, to mask any smells inside the pouch. Most ostomy companies make liquid or gel deodorants to drop into the pouch. Many people swear by TIC TAC® mints (the white ones, not other colors). Drop one or two in the pouch with every change. I've heard of people adding a spoonful of 3% hydrogen peroxide, baking soda, or minty mouthwash (the kind *without alcohol!*), or a couple of drops of peppermint oil on a cotton ball dropped into the pouch.

Breath fresheners meant to be sprayed into your mouth can also be sprayed into the pouch after emptying it or with every new pouch.

Personally, I use baby oil. Every time I empty, just before reattaching the pouch to the baseplate, I put a few squirts of baby oil into the new bag liner. It acts as a lubricant, encouraging output to slide down to the bottom, but a nice side effect is that it leaves a light, fresh smell. There are also lubricating deodorants designed just for this dual purpose and available from ostomy suppliers.

## In the toilet

Toilet sprays like POO-POURRI® or V.I.POO® are made to be spritzed into the toilet *before* anything else hits the water. The idea is that it spreads out like a film over the surface. As your output breaks through and submerges beneath it, odors are trapped under there. These products aren't specifically made for ostomates, but we're probably their best customers!

I don't do this daily, but I do carry a small bottle of toilet spray in my emergency kit for more public occasions, like when I'm using the bathroom in someone's home or on an airplane.

### In the bathroom

Keeping the bathroom smelling fresh is important for your psychological well-being. Ventilation fans are a big help. I don't have one, or even a window to crack open. So I use an automatic air freshener that emits a quick spritz every few minutes.

Make sure your discarded supplies (emptied pouches or bag liners, used wipes, etc.) are well sealed before disposal. If the sealed bags are left in a trash basket for any length of time, a couple of drops of an essential oil will help keep things even fresher.

I've lived in an all-female household for several years now, where the toilet seat remains down at all times. So I used to forget about the seamy underside of the seat until scrub-down day. But once I had an ileostomy, with all its splashy output, I quickly realized how important it was to clean under the seat frequently.

Tiny brown splashes can defy the laws of physics and find their way to the most unlikely places, like under the toilet bowl or the toe kick of a vanity. A thorough cleaning of all these nooks and crannies, particularly after a "splashy" landing, will help keep the bathroom fresh.

## Gas

It's normal for the stoma to produce gas (flatulence), which accumulates in your pouch – sometimes filling it up like a balloon.

Many foods and beverages are said to increase gas. See the *Food Tables* in Appendix A to learn which foods can cause gas, and which ones help to reduce it.

# WHAT COULD POSSIBLY GO WRONG?

Other potential causes of excess gas are drinking through a straw, chewing gum, slurping or gulping your food, not chewing well, and talking while eating. Turns out your mother was right!

Many ostomates take over the counter (OTC) gas and bloating remedies like BEANO® and GAS-X®.

Remember that people without ostomies produce a surprising amount of gas every day too. The only difference is where it comes out. When it comes out of your rectum, it dissipates into the air behind you. But when it comes from a stoma, it builds up in your pouch until it's released … right under your nose.

## Ballooning (and not the fun kind, either)

An unreleased build-up of gas will cause the pouch to inflate like a balloon. It could even inflate to the point of causing smells, leaks, or a dreaded blow-out.

Another problem with ballooning is trying to empty the contents of a pouch filled with gas, particularly if the output is watery. As soon as you open the pressurized pouch, it's liable to spew.

So how do you deal with ballooning? There are 3 options: filters, vents, and burping.

- **Filters**

    Many pouches come with filters that allow gas to escape, but trap or neutralize odor. They'll stop working if they get wet. Some claim to be waterproof; others come with stickers to place over the filter, supposedly to prevent water from coming in (when showering, bathing, swimming, etc.). A far more common problem is watery output from inside the pouch wetting the filter, or thicker output clogging it.

    However it happens, if your filter becomes wet or clogged you'll have to change to a new pouch if you want to avoid filling up with gas.

When I use pouches that come with filters, I usually keep them blocked with the stickers all the time. I don't have a high gas output and don't mind if the pouch inflates with a little gas because it makes some space for my output to drop down inside. Of course, people with a higher gas output are at more risk of ballooning if they block the filter.

Many people claim they can get at least a few days' wear out of a pouch with a filter before it clogs and/or stops working. Others say they're lucky to get one day. There are several different companies making these products, so you have lots to try out to see if you can find one that works well for you.

I use bag liners inside my pouch. The instructions say to puncture a couple of holes near the top of the liners, to allow gas to escape. You don't *need* to do that (I don't), but if you have a higher gas output, you might want to try it. It's meant to allow the gas to escape from the bag liner into the pouch and out through the filter.

- **Vents**

    Another option is to use a small vent mechanism called OSTO-EZ-VENT® – that you buy separately and attach to your pouch. This brand may not be the only externally applied vent out there but it's the only one I know of, and it's very popular.

    The vents come with detailed instructions and there are good videos online showing how to attach them. Basically, you peel off the backing and stick it on the outside of your pouch, near the top. Then you poke through a small hole in the center of the vent, making an opening into the pouch. The vent has an outside cover that you flip open to let gas escape, as needed. Some ostomates find all this a bit "fiddly." But for many others, it's a very workable solution to the problem of gas build-up. When they get a new supply of pouches and vents, they simply attach a whole batch of them at one time, assembly line fashion, so they have a good supply of vented pouches on hand, ready to go.

- **Burping the pouch**

If you have a 2-piece appliance, with or without a bag liner, you may find the easiest way to get rid of gas build-up is to burp the pouch (like a TUPPERWARE® food container). Just open it a bit at the top to let the air escape, usually with a satisfying "pffffttt," then close it up again. Voilà!

This works best with a pouch that attaches mechanically to the baseplate, by clicking or locking into place. Self-adhesive pouches may not re-adhere well to the baseplate after you've peeled the top back to burp a few times. When I used an adhesive pouch, I found I could actually completely remove and re-attach it several times, with little or no loss of adhesion. But every product is different. You won't know till you try.

If there's watery output in your pouch along with a lot of gas (in other words, if the pouch is very inflated and ready to spew), it can spray out when you burp it. Under those conditions, if you have a drainable pouch, you'd be safer to release the gas from the bottom opening while standing over a toilet.

As mentioned in the *Sleeping* section in Chapter 5, some ostomates find that their pouches inflate significantly overnight, so they wake up with a pressurized balloon on their stomach. This isn't just uncomfortable. It also poses a risk of the pouch pulling away from the baseplate or bursting if you roll over on it. The best strategy here is to reduce gas as much as possible by paying attention to what, when, and how you eat, and/or by taking anti-gas remedies before bedtime.

Some folks say they've gotten used to waking up during the night, burping or emptying their pouches, and then going right back to sleep. If you're fortunate enough to master this trick, it's a great solution to overnight ballooning.

### Abdominal discomfort

Gas isn't just a pouch problem. It can also be painful. In addition to learning what to eat and what to avoid, tips for reducing abdominal gas pains include applying a heating pad across your stomach, a light massage, exercise like walking, and hot drinks.

 **Keep in mind that if this becomes a chronic problem, or is accompanied by other symptoms you can't explain, like nausea or vomiting, maybe it's not just gas. There are many other causes of abdominal pain. Worth checking out with a doctor.**

## Constipation (colostomies)

Constipation rarely or never occurs with ileostomies because they don't produce fully formed stool. If anything, ileostomy output can be too watery. But constipation can happen if you have a colostomy. You're no more or less likely to become constipated now than you were before. The only real difference is that now you can't strain to push it out.

Some people with colostomies go a few days with little or no output, and then a day or two with more. This is their normal pattern, and it doesn't mean they're constipated. But if it isn't typical, or if it goes longer than usual or is accompanied by discomfort, then constipation should be considered.

### Symptoms

The main symptom is **minimal or no output** for an unusual length of time.

This may be accompanied by cramping and the usual symptoms of constipation. But if the pain is severe, and especially if it's accompanied by nausea or vomiting, it may be a blockage and require more serious treatment.

# WHAT COULD POSSIBLY GO WRONG?

## Causes of constipation

- A diet low in fiber
- Not drinking enough water
- Side effects of medication
- Other medical causes, which usually existed before the ostomy
- A lack of exercise

## How to avoid constipation

The goal is to bulk up the stool with fiber, drink enough fluids to soften it, keep the intestines lubricated to allow easy passage, and stimulate the GI (gastrointestinal) muscles to contract in waves, moving things along.

The two most important things to prevent constipation are fiber and water.

*[**Remember, this doesn't apply to ileostomates** because their food exits their bodies before it's formed into stool. In fact, eating too much fiber will increase their risk of blockages.* **And it may not apply to colostomates with underlying medication conditions,** *like IBD, Celiac disease, etc. – who should check with a doctor first.]*

Fiber comes in two forms – soluble and insoluble. Most fiber-rich foods contain both types and that's good, because you need both. Soluble fiber softens the stool. Insoluble fiber adds bulk. Together, they make it easier to pass through your system. Think Goldilocks. "This stool is too hard. This stool is too soft. This stool is just right!"

See the *Food Tables* (Appendix A) for ideas about what to eat, and what to avoid, to prevent and manage constipation.

Remember that **the more fiber you consume, the more water you need**. If you don't drink enough, your body will find its own water by drawing it out of your stool and this can actually *cause* constipation.

Don't eat massive amounts of fiber-rich foods in one meal. That can cause bloating. Instead, eat smaller portions throughout the day. Also, don't suddenly go fiber crazy if your body isn't used to it. Add more fiber to your diet gradually.

How much fiber you need varies with individuals, but a general rule is 20 grams a day for women and 30 grams for men. That's not too hard to achieve. Here's what about 25 grams of fiber would look like, over a typical day:

| Apple, with skin | 1 medium |
| --- | --- |
| Cooked oatmeal | 1 cup (or 250 gr) |
| Raspberries | ½ cup (or 60 gr) |
| Raw carrots | 1 cup (or 100 gr) |
| Baked beans | ¾ cup (or 175 gr) |

- OR -

| 100% whole wheat bread | 2-3 slices |
| --- | --- |
| Broccoli, cooked | ½ cup (or 75 gr) |
| Orange | 1 medium |
| Avocado | 1 medium |
| Almonds | 1 small handful |

Your body was made to poop in the morning. That's when colon contractions are most active. A good way to kick start the process is with a high fiber breakfast and a hot beverage. Any warm liquid relaxes the muscles and makes the contractions easier.

Coffee is particularly effective because it stimulates the colon. 2-3 cups a day is good. But don't go crazy. Because coffee is a natural diuretic (something that makes the body release more water, through urine), too much of it can cause dehydration and actually *make* you constipated!

Some people say that a tablespoon of vegetable oil every day may help to keep stool soft and moist, and the intestinal walls "slippery."

Keep moving. Even a daily walk can make a difference.

## What to do if you're constipated

The most important thing to do if you're constipated is to figure out why, so you can avoid it recurring or even becoming chronic. But once you're dealing with it, here are some tips that can help:

Increase your intake of fiber and fluids.

Have a warm bath or shower, or put a heating pad on your abdomen. Heat relaxes the stomach muscles.

Gently massage your abdomen and the area around your stoma.

Exercise, like walking, is helpful.

Take a natural laxative, like prune juice. Many people report that drinking a beer works as a laxative for them too.

You can try an OTC medication or supplement before resorting to stronger prescription medications. Most come in liquid or tablet form. Examples include:

- **Bulking agents**, like METAMUCIL® or BENEFIBER®. These are mild laxatives that bulk up the stool with fiber. It's often the first choice of doctors when recommending an OTC treatment for constipation.

- **Magnesium citrate** and MIRALAX® are osmotic laxatives (meaning they draw more water into the bowel and keep it there longer). This kind of laxative is often used when the stool is hard or impacted. It's usually the second choice, after trying bulking agents.

- **Senna**. This is a stimulant laxative (meaning it stimulates the muscles to squeeze harder than usual). It's often used when the stool is soft but still difficult to pass. Senna is a natural medicine that comes from the leaves of the senna plant. It's the principal ingredient in some non-prescription laxatives, like SENOKOT®.

 If your constipation becomes chronic, lasts unusually long, or causes pain, nausea, or vomiting, it's time to stop the home remedies and speak to a doctor.

# Blockages

Blockages (or "obstructions" as they're called in the medical world) can be a temporary discomfort or serious enough to require medical attention. Here's what you need to know:

### Symptoms

Like with constipation, the primary symptom is **minimal or no output** for an unusual length of time (from several hours, if that's not your norm, to a few days). Other symptoms can include:

- Watery output that has a foul smell
- Stoma looks bigger than normal
- Movement in intestines that can be heard or felt
- Burping
- Passing little or no gas
- Distended abdomen, may be firm and tender to touch
- Abdominal cramps, particularly near the stoma. Often in waves
- Sweating
- Nausea or vomiting
- Decreased urination
- Dark colored urine
- Dry mouth

# WHAT COULD POSSIBLY GO WRONG?

Blockages in the large intestine (colostomies) usually happen gradually. Those in the small intestine (ileostomies) can happen fast.

A blockage may be partial (watery output, with minimal or no stool) or total (no output at all). Cramping pains tend to be more severe in a total blockage.

 **If you have signs of dehydration, if you've had no output for an unusual length of time or an excessive amount of all-liquid output, and especially you're vomiting or in severe pain - get to the ER!**

*If you go to the ER, take the UOAA's Ileostomy Blockage Guide (Appendix C) with you. It provides helpful information for ER staff on how to treat an ileostomy blockage.*

## Causes

A blockage is pretty much like a clogged drainpipe. It can be one of two types. The first type is more common.

- **Mechanical blockage** (or "dynamic" obstruction) - This is a physical obstruction in the intestine. It might be a food blockage (more common with ileostomies), or a structural blockage like an adhesion from scar tissue.

- **Paralytic ileus** ("adynamic" obstruction, or "ileus") - This happens when the normal muscle contractions in the intestine stop (due to an infection or a few other reasons). These contractions move the contents of your bowels along their usual path. If they stop, nothing is going to move.

You can't determine yourself what kind of blockage it is. That can only be done by diagnostic tests.

## How to avoid food blockages

You have no control over structural blockages, but by controlling what you eat, you can reduce the chance of a food blockage, which is more common.

This kind of blockage can happen when food with fiber or roughage hasn't been chewed or digested properly and forms a sort of dam, blocking the passage of output.

### Ileostomates:

Your food only passes through your small intestine (where nutrients are absorbed) before exiting your body. It's never processed into regular stool because it never reaches the large intestines. Some of what you eat may even come out exactly as it went in (like corn, and slow release pills). That's why food blockages happen more frequently with ileostomies. To help prevent food blockages with ileostomies ...

- Eat a low-residue diet - with little fiber or other materials that remain after digestion. And chew, chew, chew!
- Drink plenty of water.
- Eat more frequent, smaller meals. Give your system a chance to process your food without being overwhelmed.
- See the *Food Tables* (Appendix A) for ideas about what to eat, and what to avoid.

### Colostomates:

Food blockages are far less common with colostomies, but they can still happen. So colostomates should still be careful to chew their food well, and drink plenty of water.

Though it's ok, and actually recommended, for most colostomates (like those with no underlying medical condition such as IBD) to follow a fiber-rich diet, avoid anything that may have blocked you up in the past. For instance, some people have problems with popcorn and others don't.

## What to do if you suspect a blockage (of any kind)

Whether you have an ileostomy or colostomy, if your symptoms aren't too severe, you can try some of the following techniques at home before seeking medical treatment, or until you have a chance to see your doctor. Just don't wait too long. If things don't start moving soon, seek help.

Stop eating solid foods. You want to break down the dam, not build it up.

If it's a partial blockage (only a little output, and nothing solid), drink more clear liquids. Hot drinks like tea or coffee are good. Many people find that a carbonated beverage like COKE® clears them out pretty quickly. Others swear by 100% pure red grape juice.

If it's a total blockage (no output of any kind) or if you're vomiting, don't eat or drink *anything*.

If your stoma looks swollen, you may need to cut the hole in your baseplate a little larger so you won't constrict it.

Like with constipation, heat helps relax the stomach muscles. Have a warm bath or shower, or put a heating pad on your abdomen.

Gently massage your abdomen and the area around your stoma.

Walking can help. Also, stretching exercises – ex., lie on your back, knees bent, and rock your legs from side to side. Or stretch out your torso while standing (twist from the waist, bend over, or reach your arms up over your head). The idea is to encourage your intestines to move and hopefully dislodge a small blockage.

**Ileostomates need to be especially vigilant about blockages. You can get into trouble quickly. Waiting too long can have serious consequences. If you've tried the above techniques and they haven't worked, you should seek medical help immediately.**

All medical sources warn against taking laxatives or stool softeners (OTC or prescribed) if you suspect a blockage. They can do more harm than good, and are a bad idea at any time for someone with an ileostomy.

After your blockage has been resolved, be extra careful about what you eat for a few days. Your intestines have been through the wringer and like you, they need a chance to recover.

## So which is it? - Constipation or blockage?

Both conditions can look alike in the early stages. In both cases, the first sign is usually little or no output. What you choose to do at this point can make it better or much worse, depending on whether it's actually constipation or a blockage.

So how do you know which condition to treat for? If you're passing gas, it's probably constipation – particularly if you're a colostomate. If you're not passing gas, it's more likely a blockage, particularly if your abdomen is distended. Beyond that, the best you can do is figure out all the possibilities and go with the most likely. The scenarios on the next page are examples of ostomates figuring out what they're probably dealing with. Just remember – **if you start having pain, vomiting, and/or significant nausea, stop whatever you're doing and seek medical attention!**

# WHAT COULD POSSIBLY GO WRONG?

### DANIELLE (ileostomy, food blockage)

- Danielle's had an ileostomy for several years.
- No history of any kind of blockage.
- Yesterday she came back from a cruise, where she wasn't as careful as usual about food. All that fresh tropical fruit was so tempting!
- Her stomach has been "churning" since last night.
- Her output is minimal and has an unusually strong and unpleasant odor.
- She decides it's probably a partial food blockage and follows those tips.
- If the pain gets worse or she feels nauseous, she'll call the doctor.

### KEVIN (colostomy, mechanical blockage)

- Kevin's had a colostomy for many years.
- His diet (high fiber, lots of water) hasn't changed.
- His output has been slowing down over time. He didn't even notice at first. But now he's had almost no output at all for more than a day, which is really unusual for him. And he's started to have cramps.
- He's been constipated before. This feels different.
- He suspects it's a blockage. He stops eating, applies heat, exercises, massages his abdomen, and drinks grape juice. No result.
- The next day, he consults his doctor, who sends him for tests.
- Turns out to be stenosis, a gradual narrowing of the stoma, which is easily corrected with minor surgery.

> **TERRI (colostomy, constipation)**
>
> - Terri's had a colostomy for two years. She has no underlying medical condition.
> - Her pattern is to go several days with no output and no discomfort. Then it's like the dam breaks. It starts with waves of cramps (not severe, but uncomfortable), and then over the several hours, her pouch fills up over and over, often pancaking.
> - She never thought it was constipation because when it starts, the stool isn't hard and it passes very easily.
> - Then her stoma nurse points out that this isn't normal and recommends a high fiber diet.
> - Shortly after Terri increases her fiber and water intake, she starts passing firm, well-formed stool almost every day. It *was* constipation after all!
> - She loved the cost savings and convenience of not having to change her pouch very often, but this is definitely healthier and she's going to stick to a high fiber diet.

# Diarrhea

Diarrhea obviously means watery or loose stool – much more than usual in the case of ileostomates, whose output is already pretty liquid. Colostomates can recognize diarrhea pretty easily, but ileostomates have to judge it by quantity. For most ileostomates, normal daily output is about 3–4 cups or 900 ml. That means about 6 half-filled, medium-sized pouches a day. If it's suddenly a lot more than that, and this is more than their normal volume, it's probably diarrhea.

WHAT COULD POSSIBLY GO WRONG?

### Symptoms

- Sudden onset of loose/liquid stool (more than typical for ileostomates)
- May have cramps
- If severe, may show dehydration symptoms – like dry mouth, dark urine, nausea, and feeling weak

### Causes

- Certain foods (like foods that are natural laxatives, or foods that aren't well tolerated by the individual)
- Contaminated food or water
- Digestive disorders (like IBD and celiac disease)
- Intestinal flu or bug
- Chemo or radiation therapy
- Side effect of some prescription medications
- Emotional stress, sometimes

### What to do about it

The main risks of diarrhea are dehydration and an imbalance of electrolytes.

Even if it seems counter-intuitive, drink lots of liquids.

Drink a combination of water and drinks that replenish electrolytes, like sports drinks.

- You can make your own electrolyte drink – one that includes sugar and salt … so something like a half-and-half mixture of orange juice and water, with a little salt.

- Or drink a cup of sweetened liquid, like clear sweet tea, and an hour later drink something salty, like a clear salty broth. Keep this up, switching between sweet & salty drinks every hour.

Avoid foods that worsen diarrhea. Eat those that thicken output and are high in potassium, to replace what you're losing. See the *Food Tables* (Appendix A) for examples.

An easy reminder of some good foods to eat while you have diarrhea is the **BRAT** acronym:

**B**ananas, **R**ice (white), **A**pplesauce & **T**oast (white).

 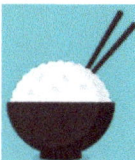  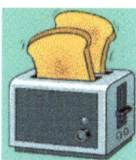

 **If diarrhea continues despite these tips, or if you develop dehydration or other symptoms like blood in your stool, stomach pain, fever, or nausea, call your doctor or go to the ER.**

# Leaks

Leaks are a pretty common problem – particularly in the early days, and particularly for ileostomates, as their output is more watery. But it can happen to any of us, at any time.

### General information

A leak is when your output doesn't go directly into your pouch, but finds another escape route – usually under the baseplate, which means it's going to come into contact with your skin. And that's the problem. Whether a small leak or a big one, it will irritate your skin if it's left sitting there, particularly if your output is watery.

> A leak can be obvious (you can see, feel, or smell it) or it can be sneaky (seeping under the baseplate and hiding out there, waiting to surprise you at your next appliance change).

Baseplates don't stick well to irritated skin. This opens the way for more leaks and more frequent changes ... damaging the skin even more and starting a vicious cycle.

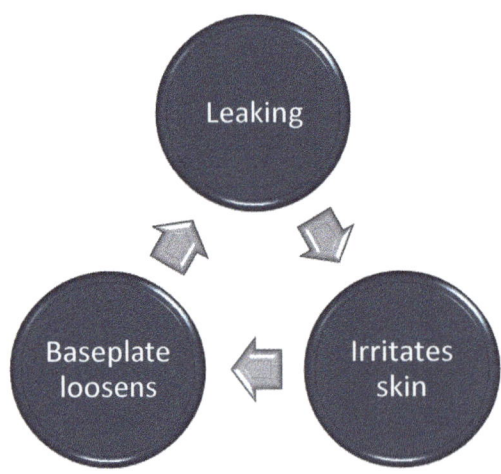

OK, that's the bad news. The good news is that because leaking is such a common problem, there are tons of products and tips out there to help you solve it.

Think of your ostomy appliance as a prison, and your output as prisoners. You're the warden. When everything goes right, the prisoners stay locked up till you're ready to release them. But you have to stay on guard. The first opportunity to make a break and they're outta there! Your job is to know when and how they're getting out, then fix it before they do too much damage or trigger a mass escape.

In a pinch, you can use a flange extender to temporarily stop a leak that's threatening to come out from under the baseplate. That's like reinforcing the fence around the prison property. It might buy you a little extra time till you can do a proper repair but it isn't a fix. You're just containing the damage. The output that's gone AWOL is going to stay under the baseplate, damaging your skin.

## Causes & remedies

In one form or another, leaking is almost always an adhesive issue. Here are several of the most common reasons why your baseplate may not be sticking well to your skin and not sealing off the stoma.

### Wrong size hole

Whether you use a pre-cut or cut-to-fit hole, it's important that it fits well around your stoma. Otherwise some output will go under the baseplate, where it can weaken the seal and cause a leak.

Make sure your pre-cut hole is the right size. If you're not sure, ask a stoma nurse to measure you.

# WHAT COULD POSSIBLY GO WRONG?

Use a pre-made template (usually supplied with baseplates) for a cut-to-fit hole. These templates have several holes, of different sizes. Hold them over your stoma, one by one, until you find the one that fits exactly. Place that template hole over the center part of your baseplate and trace the circle with a marker. Now you can cut the hole yourself. Ostomy scissors are best for this job, but I know of a few people who highly recommend seam rippers too (a tool seamstresses use to rip through stitches).

If your hole is an irregular shape, or in between the sizes on a pre-made template, you can make your own. Start with a baseplate with a hole that's the right size and shape for you (previously cut by you or your stoma nurse). Lay it on a piece of plastic or cardboard, trace the hole, and cut it out. After that, use this as a template to mark and cut future holes in your baseplates.

Another option is a moldable baseplate, where the part that goes around your stoma is made of a substance that you can stretch and mold to fit snugly, hugging your stoma like a turtleneck. This isn't a good choice if your stoma is flush, though.

Remember that your stoma hole can change size, particularly in the first several weeks after surgery. Also, if you develop a hernia or gain a lot of weight, the bulge can stretch the hole as it grows. So periodically check the size to make sure it hasn't changed.

## Stoma is retracted or flush

If the stoma doesn't stick out a little (allowing the stool to drop down into the pouch), then output can find its way under the baseplate more easily, leading to a leak.

This is what a convex baseplate is for. It presses the area around the stoma down, so it protrudes more.

**Abdomen isn't flat**

The ideal surface for a baseplate is flat. But for many of us, our abdomens have dips, dimples, creases, bumpy scars, or stitches. These can make gaps under the baseplate.

Look at the back of your baseplate after every change. You'll see where any output has seeped underneath it. That's where you may have gaps.

After washing and drying the skin, use a stoma paste (like caulking) to fill in any gaps. You can apply the paste directly to your skin, making the surface as smooth and flat as possible, or put it on the back of the baseplate so it will fill in the gap – whatever works best for you.

Don't worry about the paste touching your stoma. That's perfectly ok.

There are many paste products made for this purpose. They come in tubes, like toothpaste, or in strips, where you tear off pieces as needed. Use the minimum amount necessary to do a good job.

Tube paste usually contains alcohol, and strip pastes usually don't. The alcohol can cause a temporary burning sensation if you have broken skin. That's normal. But if it causes allergies or irritation (skin keeps burning or becomes red, blistered, or itchy), you should switch to another brand or type of paste.

If you still have stitches near the stoma, you won't want to stick the baseplate directly on top of them. If possible, cut out part of the baseplate to leave the stitches exposed. But be careful not to cut so much that the baseplate isn't well sealed all around your stoma.

### Ballooning or pancaking

A build-up of gas in the pouch (ballooning) or stool accumulating around the stoma (pancaking), can create so much pressure that it forces its way under the baseplate, creating an opening for leaks.

Release gas by burping the pouch or using pouches with a filter.

If pancaking is the problem, see the *Pancaking* section of this chapter for tips on dealing with that.

### Skin not properly prepared

For the baseplate to adhere securely, the skin should be smooth, squeaky clean, and bone dry.

Adhesive residue from the last baseplate or even excessive abdominal hair can interfere with the adhesion of the baseplate. Remove both as gently as possible.

An adhesive remover can be used to remove adhesive buildup on the skin around the stoma.

Make sure any product used on the skin, including soap and adhesive remover, is thoroughly rinsed off.

After rinsing, let the skin air dry completely or use a hair dryer on a low setting to get rid of any last traces of moisture.

### Using too much product

The less-is-more rule applies to ostomies. Baseplates are designed to stick best to bare skin, not to products.

While some products (like creams, powders, pastes, barrier sprays, etc.) may be unavoidable at times, use the bare minimum you can get away with. If you can, use no products at all.

## Skin is irritated

Baseplates don't stick well to skin that's irritated in any way. Your skin may be reacting to an adhesive used by a particular manufacturer, or it may be developing an infection or irritation for a number of reasons. See the *Skin Irritations* section of this chapter for ideas about how to treat those problems.

Meanwhile, here are some tips to help avoid output coming into contact with your skin and making it worse.

Barrier rings may be helpful. These are flat, pliable circles, almost like putty, designed to surround your stoma and form a moisture (output) barrier. The rings are sticky, so you can apply them directly on your skin, circling your stoma, or apply them to the back of your baseplate, circling the hole, before placing it on your skin. They're also stretchy, so you can stretch them to fit exactly around the stoma.

Stoma collars or "stoma hats" are designed to encourage output to flow directly through a kind of cylinder/spout and drop into the pouch without touching the skin. They're applied under the baseplate and the cylinder protrudes out through the hole in the baseplate.

Many companies make protective sheets that act as a barrier between your skin and your baseplate. These are thin, flexible sheets with an adhesive backing. You place one around your stoma, generally by cutting a hole in it, using your template. Or cut it into any shape you need if you only want to cover one area. The baseplate is then placed on top, adhering to the protective sheet (and not to your skin).

WHAT COULD POSSIBLY GO WRONG?

# Blowouts

This is a general term for epic pouch failure, from any cause, resulting in the contents spilling out. It's the stuff of ostomy nightmares, and can also be the subject of some hilarious stories (blowouts tend to be much funnier in hindsight). Ostomates rarely get together without swapping blowout horror stories.

### General information

There are many causes of blowouts. Your pouch can fill up with gas or output to the point that it's pushed off, or leak so much that it loosens the baseplate, or the bottom of your drainable pouch might suddenly open and spill its contents down your leg and onto the floor. That sort of thing.

Sometimes it's the result of an accident, like a baseplate being yanked off by an exuberant dog. But often we can look back and see where we might have been a little more vigilant. Like being too tired to empty a half-filled pouch during the night, or forgetting to properly secure the bottom of a drainable pouch. Lesson learned.

It can happen anywhere – in bed, in a board meeting, or in the grocery store. The only common element is a mess. And probably swearing.

That's why we carry emergency kits and keep changes of clothes at the office or in the car.

If you're prone to blowouts, a waterproof mattress pad can be a lifesaver. So can incontinence pads that go on top of the bottom sheet.

Be prepared but not scared. Although it's not uncommon, there are people who've never had a blowout. Ever. Not even after decades with an ostomy.

## Cleanup

If it does happen, don't panic or be hard on yourself. As all ostomates know, s***t happens. Just focus on cleaning up. Have a shower. Change your appliance. And then tackle the debris field – clothing, floor, sheets, furniture, the dog, whatever got soiled.

Clothing and sheets can be cleaned by rinsing off anything you can, then soaking for several hours in cold water.

You can pre-treat with a stain remover (like a mixture of 1 part lemon juice or vinegar and 2 parts water, or a paste of cream of tartar and water), and/or add detergents containing enzymes to the soaking water. An enzyme called protease is best for protein stains. It's found in laundry products like TIDE® Liquid Coldwater detergent, BIZ® stain remover, and WISK® detergent.

> Enzymes in meat tenderizers also work because they're used to break down proteins. Make a paste with <u>unseasoned</u> meat tenderizer and water, apply it to the stain, and let sit for a half hour before the next step.

After pre-treating and/or soaking, wash in cold or warm water with some bleach added. Chlorine bleach is ok for white fabrics, and an oxygen bleach like OXY CLEAN® is best for colors. You can add baking soda (bicarbonate of soda) or washing soda to boost the effect of either bleach.

Don't use chlorine bleach and a detergent with enzymes together. It won't do any harm, but the chlorine deactivates the enzymes, so you should use them separately (like one in the soak, and one in the wash). Oxygen bleach is ok to mix with enzymes.

Drying washed fabrics in direct sunlight will help bleach out stains even more.

Pet stain removers can work well on carpets and upholstery, and even mattresses.

## Pancaking

This is when thick, pasty stool accumulates around the stoma instead of falling down into the pouch. As more output is produced, it can start pushing under the baseplate because it has nowhere else to go. If not caught and corrected in time, this can cause leaks and skin irritation.

Pancaking generally happens for one of two reasons, and often a combination of both:

- The stool is too pasty
- The pouch isn't open enough for stool to drop down into it

To "bulk up" stool, increase your intake of insoluble fiber. Bran cereal, dates & figs, lentils, nuts, and avocados are particularly rich in insoluble fiber. Bulking agents like METAMUCIL® or BENEFIBER® can be helpful here too, if you have trouble getting enough fiber through your diet. *[Note: This doesn't apply to ileostomates, who shouldn't eat a high fiber diet. And remember, ostomates with underlying medical conditions should always consult with a doctor or registered dietician before making changes to their diet).*

If you're increasing your fiber, whether through diet or a bulking agent, remember to increase your water intake too. This might sound odd, since the goal is to make the stool less pasty, but it's important. Without extra water, the stool can become too hard. You don't want to cross the line into constipation!

You also want to make it easier for the stool to drop away from your stoma and down into the pouch. Sometimes your pouch can stick to itself, like plastic cling wrap, leaving no space for the output to drop into. There are a few tricks to deal with that.

When applying a new pouch or bag liner, blow air into it to make sure it's not stuck together.

Squeeze a little oil into the pouch opening (or the bag liner after it's inside the pouch), and rub it around to coat the inside, from top to bottom. You can buy a lubricating deodorant made especially for this purpose, or use baby oil. I've even heard of some people spraying cooking oil into the pouch. Whatever you use, make sure it doesn't get on the flange, as this could interfere with the seal of the pouch.

Pouches with filters allow gas to escape. That's a good thing if you have excessive gas. But if it works too well, it can be almost like a vacuum, sucking air out of the pouch and making it stick to itself. If this is happening, try blocking the filters with the little stick-on tabs that usually come with the pouches.

Another way to keep the pouch open is to drop a wad of wet toilet paper into the bottom. This creates a little space at the bottom of the pouch. It's not a perfect solution, but anything's worth a try.

Some ostomy supply companies offer small foam blocks to place inside the pouches, keeping the sides apart. These are called "stoma bridges."

Excessive pressure from tight clothes or tummy wraps can flatten the pouch and keep output from falling into it. Try loosening them up a little to see if it helps.

Stoma guards are another helpful product. They're fairly rigid and function like athletic cups. Although principally designed to protect the stoma from injury (like in sports or other physical activities), stoma guards are also great for preventing the pouch - and therefore your output - from being squished and flattened by tight clothes or binders.

Personally, I had a lot of pancaking with a colostomy until I started using bag liners. Once inserted into the pouch, I shove my fingers down into the liner to make sure it's open and roomy. Then I squirt a little baby oil into the opening.

Everyone's different. What works like magic for one person may not work at all for another. Try a few different techniques to find the best pancaking solution for you.

WHAT COULD POSSIBLY GO WRONG?

## Skin Irritations

Healthy skin is a critical issue for ostomates. Irritated skin can be very painful and difficult to treat, and it can interfere with the adhesion of baseplates. Check your skin with every change. And be ready to swing into action when something's not right.

Remember that skin irritation is a medical issue and best treated by a medical professional. New ostomates in particular should consult with their physician or stoma nurse at the first sign of a problem under the baseplate. At the other end of the spectrum, people who've had ostomies for years, even decades, are generally familiar with the skin problems they're prone to. And they can become pretty knowledgeable about how to treat them. They usually know when it's an issue they can deal with themselves and when to call in the professionals.

The following explanations about symptoms and treatments are intended to help you be informed, wherever you are on the ostomy spectrum. The more you know, the less likely that a small problem will escalate into something more serious.

### Symptoms

If you have one or more of these symptoms, it's a sign of irritation.

- Redness
- Itching
- Burning
- Small bumps
- Inflammation
- Dampness
- Bleeding (other than normal, mild bleeding from the stoma when wiped)
- Raw, weepy skin or blisters

## Causes & treatments

Skin irritations can appear for many different reasons. But these are four of the most common causes:

### 1. Mechanical irritation

This is an irritation or trauma due to external forces. It means the skin is being damaged by some kind of action or exposure to something damaging – which is good news, because you can take steps to correct it. These are the most common types of mechanical irritation:

- **Frequent appliance changes**

    Changing your appliance too often (like a few times a day versus once every few days) can strip away skin without giving it time to heal in between.

    There are a number of reasons why you might be changing your baseplate too often. You have to identify and treat the *cause* (leaking? allergy to the adhesive? irritated skin?) before you can change the *effect* (frequent changes). Consult with a stoma nurse if you need help. Hopefully, after you've solved the underlying problem, you'll be measuring your change intervals in days, not hours.

- **Being too rough on your skin**

    Washing the skin around your stoma too harshly will damage it. Wash the area gently with a soft cloth or tissue. This is no time or place for scrubbing. Yeeouch!

    Pulling off the baseplate too roughly can be harmful too. Push the skin down with one hand while you gently remove the baseplate with the other, working your way around. Think of it as pushing the skin away from the baseplate, rather than peeling the baseplate off the skin. Use an adhesive remover if it doesn't come away easily.

# WHAT COULD POSSIBLY GO WRONG?

- **Pressure ulcers**

    These are sores that can develop from the pressure of convex baseplates, which are often necessary for stomas that are flush or retracted. It doesn't happen to everyone, but unfortunately it does happen, particularly if you have a peristomal hernia.

     **This is no time for home remedies. See a medical professional like a stoma nurse to treat the ulcers and find a workable solution so it won't keep happening.**

    Pressure ulcers begin as a reddened area, so they're easy to miss and can be mistaken for any other irritation. The skin eventually thickens and is more recognizable as an ulcer, or open sore.

    These ulcers are not generally around the base of the stoma, but are located under a rigid part of the baseplate, like the part of a convex baseplate that presses into the skin.

## 2. Contact dermatitis

This is a skin rash caused by contact with something that causes an irritant or allergic reaction. There are two types:

- **Irritant dermatitis** can happen when your skin is repeatedly exposed to fecal matter under the baseplate (versus an allergic reaction to a chemical or product). This reaction is usually quicker to develop, and when it does, it can burn and sting. The skin may look red and moist.

> The output from an ileostomy is particularly corrosive to the skin. It's alkaline (not acidic, as many people think). But that's worse. It contains digestive enzymes, so when it's left on the skin it actually starts to digest it.

# Skin irritations

This can happen for several reasons – like leaking, the wrong size hole, or a stoma that's flush or retracted. **Address the cause.** Speak to a stoma nurse, stop the leaking, correct the hole size, investigate convex baseplates, whatever it takes to keep your skin clean and safe from leaks.

**Meanwhile, treat the damaged skin.** After gently rinsing and drying the skin, cover the affected area with a very light dusting of stoma powder (to absorb moisture), then top that with a barrier spray or barrier wipe to seal it in. If you use a wipe, daub it on. Don't actually wipe across the skin, or you might wipe the powder right off.

If this doesn't do the trick, you can apply multiple layers. First the powder, then barrier spray or wipes. Repeat for 2-3 layers, allowing the barrier layer to dry thoroughly before putting on more powder. This is called "crusting" and is best done if the irritation is around the perimeter of the stoma, not over a large area.

Instead of a barrier spray marketed specifically for ostomies, you could try a liquid bandage. This comes in spray form, and serves the same purpose. And it's available OTC at pharmacies.

A remedy that's frequently used is calamine lotion, to soothe and dry out damp, irritated skin. If you pour a little into a saucer and let it become pasty (less liquid), it's easier to dab onto your skin. Apply sparingly and as always, let it dry completely before sealing with a spray. This is a good choice for a large area of irritation.

Whatever type of product you use on the skin around the stoma, always top it with a barrier spray or wipe before applying the baseplate. Just make sure any excess powder is dusted off first, and any cream has dried or been thoroughly absorbed into your skin ... then the barrier spray or wipe, then the baseplate.

A lot of ostomates swear by tincture of benzoin. This is an OTC adhesive product often used to treat damaged skin (e.g., to protect the skin from contact with an irritant, and/or to help the baseplate adhere longer). Some ostomates use this instead of a barrier spray. Dab it on with a cotton ball or swab. Allow to dry for several minutes and become tacky before putting on the baseplate. You should be aware, though, that this product contains alcohol and may burn or sting irritated skin. So try it on a small area first.

- **Allergic dermatitis** means your body is actually allergic to a product. The reaction might take a long time to develop.

  It may be a reaction to particular brand of baseplate (usually to the adhesive used by that brand) or to a product you're using – even if you've been using the same brand or product for a long time with no problem.

  Red, itchy or burning skin, sometimes progressing to blisters or welts, often indicates allergic dermatitis, particularly if it covers an area that exactly matches where the product or baseplate was applied.

  Trial and error is the only way to find another product your skin will tolerate. Get your hands on as many samples from different companies as you can. Test them on other parts of your body, leaving them in place for 48 hours. If your skin starts to get irritated before that, remove the product and wash the skin well. But if you make it through 48 hours without a reaction, it's probably safe to use it around your stoma.

  Don't forget it's not just baseplate adhesives that can trigger an allergic reaction – it may be a wipe, spray, powder, paste, ring, or any other ostomy product or accessory. It may even be soap if you're using that to wash the area (in which case, stop using soap and switch to just plain water).

Some people react to the alcohol that's in many products. Alcohol will often sting for a few seconds if the product is placed on broken skin, but if the stinging persists beyond that, try to find a non-alcohol substitute.

Many folks whose skin reacts to ostomy products manage well by using barrier sprays or wipes with every change. For them, this is all they need to lay down a protective barrier between their skin and baseplate.

Doctors often prescribe a topical steroid ointment to deal with the irritation while you're on the hunt for a product you don't react to. These creams can interfere with the adhesion of baseplates though, so be sure to seal them with a barrier spray. You can also dust the area with stoma powder before the spray.

Another option is to use a steroid nasal spray, asthma pump, ear drops, or eye drops that contain corticosteroids – but are water-based. The idea is that you can get the steroids onto your skin without it being in a cream or ointment. You'll still need a doctor's prescription, but it's a good temporary treatment for skin that's become inflamed due to contact dermatitis.

## 3. Infections

There are two main types of infections ostomates need to watch out for – yeast/fungal and hair follicle inflammation. The first one is more common.

- **Yeast/fungal infection**

    A yeast or fungus called *Candida albicanis* is normally found in your intestines. That's ok. But if it gets out (like with leaking), it can really take hold in the warm, dark, moist environment under your baseplate. It usually appears as red, shiny, flat patches with small, raised bumps

## WHAT COULD POSSIBLY GO WRONG?

that may look like blisters or pimples, and can cluster together to form a rash. Unlike an allergic reaction, the irritation may extend beyond the baseplate, or only cover part of the area under the baseplate.

This kind of infection is best treated with anti-fungal powders and creams. Your doctor can prescribe one (like Nystatin or DIFLUCAN®), or you can try some of these OTC treatments that have worked well for many ostomates:

- Wash the area with a zinc-based shampoo, like HEAD & SHOULDERS® (classic formula, without a built-in conditioner). Lather and then rinse really well.

- Swab the infected area with gentian violet, an antiseptic solution (antibacterial, antifungal) widely available in drug stores. Several medical journals and wound care nurses have recommended it for fungal or yeast infections. It's been used for a long time in Asia, the Middle East, Africa, etc., to help with wound healing ... and as a dye. So apply it with a cotton swab to avoid staining your hands. It will paint your skin purple temporarily, but if you put it on an open sore it might cause a permanent purple tattoo. Because it's water-based, it dries thoroughly, unlike creams and ointments, and that's good for baseplate adhesion. Apply a 1% solution of gentian violet to the affected area 1-3 times a day for a few days. If you see no improvement, try something else.

- Apply an anti-fungal powder used for athlete's foot, like DESENEX®. Use this instead of a regular stoma powder while you have a fungal infection. As always, don't go overboard. Use a minimum amount. Brush off any excess powder and follow with a barrier spray to seal it in.

- Another product many ostomates swear by is a zinc oxide cream like BOUDREAUX'S BUTT PASTE® (used for diaper rash), which has a high level of zinc. Apply the paste and let it sit on the infected skin for several minutes or longer. Then gently wipe or wash it off, make sure the area is very dry, and apply whatever powder you're using. Because this cream is so thick, it can be hard to completely remove and this can interfere with the adhesion of your baseplate. You may have to change your appliance more frequently for a few days (reapplying more paste each time). But once the reddened skin has cleared up, you can go back to your usual routine.

Keeping the area dry is important. This can be a challenge in hot, humid weather. If you think you can count on your stoma to behave, give your skin a chance to breathe. Leave it exposed to the air and light for a while with every change, before applying a product or baseplate.

- **Hair follicle inflammation**

Simply removing the baseplate can inflame hair follicles, but people who have to shave their abdomens to get a better seal on their baseplate are at more risk for this. A Staph or fungal infection can take hold, often appearing as small red pinpoints at the base of hairs.

It's usually recommended to start with an antifungal treatment. If that doesn't seem to be working, then switch to an antibacterial powder.

It's better to cut your abdominal hair than shave it. If you do shave, do it in the direction the hair's growing, not against it. Use warm water, not shaving cream. If you're concerned about nicking your stoma, hold a cardboard toilet paper tube or empty prescription bottle over it for protection. Using an electric shaver is another option, and I've even heard of some folks doing laser treatments to remove abdominal hair.

## 4. Bag just won't stick!

Occasionally, for no apparent reason, a particular brand of baseplate won't adhere well to your skin. You've ruled out skin irritation and allergy. You're not using too much product. You're doing everything right. But no luck. This isn't common, but everyone's skin chemistry is different. You and your baseplate may just be incompatible.

Try samples of baseplates from other companies. You might find one that adheres well.

If other baseplates don't stick either, then a spray adhesive is worth a try. It also comes in liquid form and in wipes. Do a skin test first, on some other part of your body, to make sure you don't react to it (like burning or itching or turning red). If it's a go, then apply one layer of adhesive to clean, dry skin, in the area the baseplate will cover. Let it air dry for a few minutes before putting on the baseplate. The skin should feel sticky or tacky, not wet.

- These adhesives aren't recommended with 1-piece appliances - probably because they have to be changed (pulled off the skin) more often, and that could cause mechanical irritation.
- Use adhesive removers to remove the baseplate.

You could try a barrier sheet (a plastic film with an adhesive backing that goes on top of your skin, and under the baseplate). The baseplate might stick better to the sheet than to you.

An ostomy belt can help keep baseplates secure and tight, particularly convex ones, which should press down into your skin a bit. Attach one end of the belt to each side of the baseplate and tighten snugly around your waist. But not *too* tight. You should be able to slip a couple of fingers underneath it.

Flange extenders are another option. They're basically straight, C-shaped, or Y-shaped tapes that you apply around the edges of your baseplate. They literally "extend" the baseplate and add extra adhesion.

> Ostomy belts and flange extenders help baseplates stick to your skin better. Just make sure you're not trapping leaks under there or you'll soon have a whole new problem!

## Stoma issues

We ostomates are a funny bunch. We look at photos of other people's stomas and say things like "Ooh, that's a pretty one" and "I have stoma envy!" Much like in a beauty pageant, a winning stoma would be the perfect size, shape, and height (length), and not make loud, embarrassing farts. But let's face it – most of us are going to be runners-up, for a variety of reasons.

**Size & shape** – By size, I mean the dimension of your stoma opening, and the size (or girth) of the stoma poking through it. By shape, I mean whether your opening is a perfect circle, or some other shape, like an oval. There's no such thing as a standard size or shape. What's important to know is what's normal for you, not what's normal for anyone else. Any change in *your* normal should be noted. The most common changes you might see are:

- **Changes during surgery recovery** – Immediately after surgery, your stoma will most likely be swollen. Because you've never seen a stoma before, it may not look swollen, but expect that it will decrease in size over the next 6-8 weeks. Then it should pretty much stabilize. During this recovery period, measure the dimension of your stoma frequently when you change your appliance, in case you need to adjust the hole in your baseplate.

# WHAT COULD POSSIBLY GO WRONG?

- **Stoma opening grows** – Sometimes the opening for your stoma can get bigger. This is often caused by a hernia, pregnancy, or weight gain – anything that increases the size of your abdomen and stretches the skin. We're not talking about dramatic changes in size here, but even a tiny change can affect how exactly the baseplate fits around the stoma. If the opening in your abdomen becomes bigger than the hole in your baseplate, then output can seep underneath, causing skin irritations, leaks, and/or problems with the baseplate sticking on your skin. If you start having any of these problems, check if your opening has enlarged. If so, re-measure and adjust the hole in your baseplate.

- **Stoma swelling** – Many stomas swell at times and then go back to normal. This usually means there's a buildup of pressure from the inside, like a bowel movement about to push through. But it could also be a warning sign of a blockage.

**Length** – Typically, a stoma sticks out a little. But it could be flush with the surface of your skin, or even sink in below the surface. That's called a retracted stoma. If it sticks out more than an inch (2.5 cm), it's a prolapsed stoma. Whether it's an innie or an outie, both can be managed conservatively if it isn't too extreme. Otherwise, it can be fixed with surgery.

**Flush or retracted stoma** – The purpose of a stoma is to protrude out from your abdomen enough that the output can drop down neatly into your pouch. If it's level with your skin or sinks in below that, you can have problems with leaking, seepage, or pancaking.

A flush or retracted stoma can often be managed with a convex baseplate. This kind of baseplate has a rigid, circular indentation in the center that fits around the hole in your abdomen, pushing down around the hole so your stoma will stick out a little. You can get a light, regular, or deep convex baseplate – meaning how shallow or deep the indentation is, depending on your need.

The deeper the convexity, the more pressure you'll need to keep it pressed into your stomach. Wearing an ostomy belt that hooks into tabs on the side of your baseplate or pouch can help to keep it snug. Flange extenders can also help keep the baseplate stuck on well.

Use the minimum convexity you can get away with. The more pressure against the skin around your stoma, particularly from a rigid appliance, the greater the risk of developing pressure ulcers.

**Prolapsed stoma** – This can be caused by pressure from inside your body, like chronic coughing or sneezing, heavy lifting, weight gain, pregnancy, or a tumor. It can also happen as a result of an over-sized hole made in your abdomen during the surgery. It's more common with temporary loop stomas (either colostomy or ileostomy) than permanent end stomas.

Some prolapsed stomas change, sticking out more when you're standing and going back to normal when you're lying down. This is ok, but you should check that the stoma doesn't rub against the hole in the baseplate as it moves in and out. You won't feel this, because the stoma has no nerve endings, so you have to watch for symptoms – like bleeding or a white or yellow line on the stoma where it's been rubbing. If this is happening, you could switch to a moldable baseplate, which has no hard edges around the hole.

Whether your prolapsed stoma stays out all the time or is more mobile, the first thing to do is have a stoma nurse look at it, and decide on treatment together. **Conservative management techniques** include:

- Lying down to relax the stomach muscles and reduce the abdominal pressure, then very gently pressing on the stoma to encourage it to go back inside. Make sure you have a stoma nurse teach you how to do this first!

- If the prolapsed stoma is swollen, an ice pack (wrapped in a towel) can help reduce the swelling so it will retract. Keep the pouch on, and don't do it for more than 5 minutes at a time. Remember that if it's frequently swollen, you might need to increase the size of the hole in your baseplate.

- This next tip sounds crazy, but I've read many medical articles and reports from people who do it, all insisting that it works. Put sugar on it. I swear!! Regular, granulated sugar. Sprinkle several spoonfuls on your prolapsed or swollen stoma, leave it on for 20–30 minutes, and it will draw out excess fluid, often shrinking the stoma enough that it can retract. It's much like sprinkling sugar on sliced strawberries. It acts as a dessicant, drawing out the water. Keep a lot of gauze around the area. This can be messy. Like with strawberries, there's going to be a sugary syrup left behind.

- There are specialized pouches, belts, and stoma guards designed to protect prolapsed stomas from external trauma. Again, consult with your stoma nurse to learn what products might work best for your particular situation.

In most cases, there's no danger in having a prolapsed stoma. It's really more of an inconvenience. But occasionally, **problems can arise that require medical treatment**.

- Watch for changes in the color of your prolapsed stoma. If it becomes dark red or purple, or changes to a very pale pink, it could mean a problem with the blood supply to the stoma.

- A poor blood supply can also cause small white or pale yellow patches (ischemic ulcers).

- A third sign of trouble is a change in your stoma's temperature (i.e., instead of being body temperature, it feels cool).

- Also watch out for any change in how your stoma is producing output, particularly if it's reduced, which may be a sign of a blockage.

Stoma issues

If you notice any of these symptoms, have it checked out by your stoma nurse or surgeon. If surgery is required, they might "re-size" your stoma or "re-site" it (move it to another location on your abdomen).

**Color** – Your stoma should be the usual rosy red, moist, and shiny – like the inside of your mouth. This means it's getting a good, healthy blood supply. As mentioned above, any unusual change in its color should be checked out with a doctor.

Remember we're not talking about the color of your output here. That can often be an unusual color – most often because of something you've eaten. But that won't affect the color of your stoma.

**If your stoma becomes pale**, it means it's not getting enough blood supply. This can happen if the baseplate hole is too small. If so, change baseplates and cut a larger hole.

 **If you're sure the hole isn't too small, or color isn't restored after you enlarge the hole, go to your doctor or the ER. It could mean a blockage, an internal "pinching" of the intestine, an iron deficiency, or some other condition that needs treatment.**

**If your stoma turns dusky blue, dark brown, purple, or black**, you should seek medical advice right away. This can be a sign of necrosis (which literally means the death of tissue). In the case of a stoma, it can happen if the blood flow to or from the stoma is restricted or cut off. The necrosis can be mild and limited to a small part of the stoma, or severe and more extensive. Treatment depends on the severity.

 **The most important thing is to seek medical help immediately if you think this may be happening.**

# Granulomas

### What are they?

Granulomas are tiny red bumps that can appear on the stoma but are more often around the edge of the stoma, where it joins the skin. They can be crumbly and might bleed easily because there are a lot of capillaries (little blood vessels) in there. They're really just nodules of tissue.

### What causes them?

White blood cells accumulate in an area of injury, where their role is to remove bacteria and other microscopic debris that might prevent healing or cause infection. That's a good thing. But sometimes, they "over heal," like white blood cells on steroids, and they form these tiny overgrowths of tissue.

Obviously, the granulomas started as a response to some kind of injury. For example, it might be from the skin being irritated by overly forceful cleaning, an allergic reaction to your appliance, the baseplate rubbing around the stoma because the hole is too small, or the stoma rubbing up against the pouch because your clothes or belt are pressing against it. The formation of granulomas might also be a delayed reaction to sutures from your surgery (even if it was a long time ago). No-one seems to understand why granulomas only form occasionally, in response to these common types of injury or irritation. That's still a mystery.

### Treatment

By themselves, granulomas are harmless. More of a nuisance, really. If they're not bothering you, you can live with them forever, and many people do. But sometimes granulomas can be uncomfortable or painful or too big, and if they bleed too much they can cause baseplate adhesion problems. This is definitely something to discuss with your physician or stoma nurse – first to get a firm diagnosis of granulomas, and then to develop a treatment plan.

- It might be enough just to eliminate the aggravating factors (e.g., by cleaning more gently, wearing looser clothing, or putting a lubricating product in your pouch to reduce rubbing against the stoma).

- Medical treatment often involves applying a corticosteroid or cauterizing the granulomas with silver nitrate (chemically burning them to destroy the tissue and reduce their size). That's not as bad as it sounds. Cauterizing is often used for other things like getting rid of unwanted warts or skin tags. If that doesn't help or if the granulomas keep returning, they're sometimes removed surgically under a local anesthetic.

# Hernias

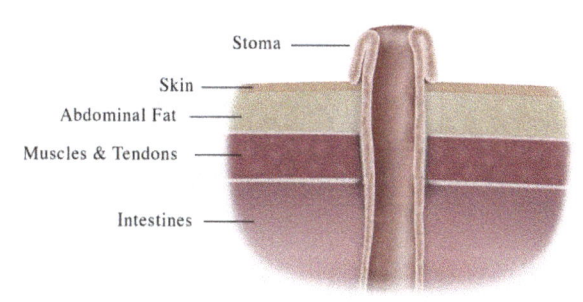

To create your stoma, the surgeon made an incision in your abdomen and created a passageway for a portion of your intestine to reach your tummy. It first passes through the membrane that contains your intestines, then through layers of muscles and tendons, then through the fatty layer beneath your skin, and finally out through an opening in the skin.

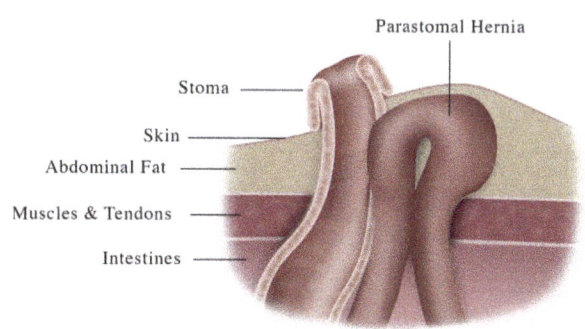

The muscles around the stoma generally support it. But sometimes the edges of the stoma pull away from the muscles, enlarging the opening and allowing more intestines to push through – like two people comically trying to squeeze through a narrow doorway (when only one of them was invited). The resulting bulge is the first sign of a parastomal hernia, which literally means "hernia around the stoma."

Once one uninvited guest has pushed through the doorway, you can be sure that more will follow. Remember that there are about 25 feet or 7½ meters of intestines squeezed into a relatively small space. That's a lot of internal pressure. So it makes sense that the intestines are going to want to push out through any small opening.

A hernia usually starts off pretty small and tends to get bigger over time, as more intestines push through the opening, enlarging it even more.

You can also develop an incisional hernia where a previous stoma was closed. The incision closing the original opening in the abdominal muscles can re-open at some point after surgery. Again, intestines will probably push through that gap and form a hernia.

### How common are hernias?

Short answer: very.

It's one of the most common complications of ostomies.

There are a lot of different numbers floating around, even from solid medical sources. But generally, most report that over time, up to about 50% of colostomates and 30% of ileostomates will develop a hernia.

John Byron Gathright, Jr., MD, Past President of the American Society of Colon & Rectal Surgeons, has been quoted as saying *"It doesn't matter if God himself made your ostomy. If you have it long enough, you have a 100% risk of a parastomal hernia."* Read that carefully, though. It doesn't mean 100% of ostomates *will* develop a hernia, but 100% of them are *at risk* for it. And that's bad enough!

## Causes

The main cause of hernias is strain – anything that increases pressure within the abdomen. Of course this includes lifting and strenuous physical activity, but also coughing and sneezing. Even strenuous laughing can do it. This is especially true in the weeks and months just after surgery. Remember all those intestines squeezed into a small space, under a lot of internal pressure, looking for a way to come out? You don't want to add to that internal pressure, especially when the opening is trying to heal itself and seal shut.

> Be careful! I've heard of hernias developing in surprising ways – from salsa dancing to straining to get out of a low car.

If you've made it a year or more post-surgery with no hernia, your odds are looking better. It's still possible to get one, but it would take more. Like heavy lifting could still do it, but a belly laugh? ... not so much.

Sometimes a post-surgical infection can result in a hernia too, but this isn't nearly as common.

## Risk factors

These risk factors increase the odds of developing a hernia because they weaken your body's resistance to abdominal strain.

- Overweight (probably the biggest risk factor)
- Female
- Over 60
- Smoking (weakens connective tissue)
- Chronic constipation
- Poor nutrition
- Some medications (like corticosteroids)

# WHAT COULD POSSIBLY GO WRONG?

- Pre-existing medical conditions (including diabetes, high blood pressure, cancer, inflammatory bowel disease, lower serum albumin levels, and advanced liver disease with ascites)
- Previous abdominal surgeries (Caesareans, previous hernia repairs, etc.)

## Complications

A hernia may never present any problems or symptoms other than an unsightly bulge. But because complications can arise in any of the following areas, even after years, it's good to stay watchful.

> Once a hernia has started, it will almost always increase in size over time. The bigger it grows and the longer you have it, the more risk of complications. It will never simply "go away."

- **Baseplate attachment** – A hernia usually makes a pronounced bulge in your abdomen. It's not as easy to attach a baseplate securely to a round and maybe uneven surface as it is to a flat surface. That's why a concave baseplate can be a good choice here. Also, if the hernia is large enough, it might mean you can't see your stoma any more, making it more difficult to attach the appliance.

- **Stoma shape** – The increasing bulge can stretch your stoma opening. This might mean switching from a baseplate with a perfectly round, pre-cut hole to one where you have to cut your own hole, in your own unique shape. This shape can change if your hernia reduces when you lie down and increases when you stand up (some hernias change with posture; some don't).

- **Stoma size** – The hernia might stretch the stoma opening to a larger size – still round, but bigger. If you don't notice this slight change and don't increase the size of your baseplate hole, it can lead to output seeping under the baseplate and irritating your skin.

- **Fragile skin** – The larger the hernia, the more your skin is being stretched. If it's stretched too much, it can become more fragile and easily irritated.

- **Stoma functioning** – A hernia can change how stool passes through your bowels. This could be anything from constipation to diarrhea.

- **Irrigation** – If you irrigate, a hernia might make it more difficult. This depends very much on the positioning of the herniated intestines.

- **Stoma retraction** – As the bulge increases, the stoma can become retracted. This can make leaking more likely. You may have to switch from a flat or concave baseplate to a convex one.

- **Stoma prolapse** – The opposite of stoma retraction. It means your stoma is protruding out of your abdomen more than normal. It can happen with or without a hernia, but because it's literally being pushed out from inside, it frequently co-occurs with a hernia. In extreme cases, it can require surgery.

- **Incarceration** – Often the intestines forming the hernia can be pushed back into place inside the intestinal wall or go back naturally, at least partway, when you're lying down. This doesn't mean the hernia's gone, of course, just that some intestines are slipping in and out of the opening in the abdominal wall with changes in posture, making the hernia slightly bigger and smaller. But sometimes the intestines can become "trapped" out there, and don't go back inside even when gently pushed. This means they're incarcerated. While these intestines won't go back inside, more can come out over time and become incarcerated too (i.e., the hernia can keep growing). This can lead to what's called "loss of domain" – see below.

- **Loss of domain** – This means more of the intestines are now outside the abdominal cavity than inside it. The loss of domain can be so significant that a hernia repair can no longer be done, or at least not without significant risk. Basically, you don't want to get to this point. So if you have a large hernia, check in with your doctor or surgeon regularly to make sure it's not getting *too* big.

- **Strangulation** – A portion of the intestine that's herniated can become twisted or kinked. Fortunately, it's not all that common. This is the most serious potential complication and often requires emergency surgery. There could be symptoms like pain and blockage, but the first thing you notice might be a change in appearance – particularly in color.

 If your stoma changes from a healthy red to a dark purple or black color, with or without pain (and with or without a hernia), it's definitely time to go to the ER.

## Prevention of a hernia

Take heart. There are many things you can do to reduce your risk of developing a hernia. You just have to be pro-active about it.

### Before ostomy surgery:

If physically possible and if you have enough time to make a difference, do exercises (like Pilates) to build up your core abdominal muscles.

I know this is easy to say, but if you're overweight, try to lose as much as you can before surgery (while keeping up your nutrition). Every little bit helps.

Stop smoking, even temporarily. Now don't roll your eyes at me, smokers. I'm one of you. Believe me, I know how hard it is! Just remember that the longer you can stop or at least cut down as much as possible, the more likely your incision will "take." Even a few weeks can make a difference.

Talk to a stoma nurse about getting a hernia belt to wear after surgery. OK, if you're a non-smoking 25-year old male fitness freak with rock hard abs, and swear you won't lift anything heavier than a Chinese noodle for the next 12 months, you might be able to skip this. But many surgeons don't even suggest it to patients at *high* risk for hernias! Bottom line: if you think you're at any risk, don't wait for someone to suggest it, because by then it may be too late. Make it your business to get a hernia belt yourself. It's a very small inconvenience for a very BIG gain.

There are other support garments on the market, like support briefs and waistbands, and abdominal binders. Like hernia belts, these all help to support the abdomen, though not as much.

## After ostomy surgery:

Smoking after surgery reduces the oxygen in your tissues (among other things), prolonging recovery and increasing the risk of infection. Even after the wound looks like it's healed on the outside, it continues healing for up to a year on the inside. Smoking can interfere with that process – increasing your chances of developing a hernia. So the longer you can stay off cigarettes post-surgery, the better.

If you have a hernia belt or other support garment, start wearing it as soon as you can. And not just if you're going to lift something. You should wear it all day, only taking it off for bathing and sleeping. If you have a chronic cough, you might even want to sleep in it too. Do this for at least 6 months. Personally, I'd do it for a year.

Remember that the goal is to support your abdominal muscles, not constrict them. Don't make it *too* tight. You know those pictures of Victorian ladies cinching in their waists until they can't breathe? Not that.

Even if you're wearing a belt or support garment, do everything you can to **avoid abdominal strain**.

- Press a pillow or folded blanket, or even just your hands, over the stoma area when you cough or sneeze. If you can do anything to reduce coughing or sneezing, this is the time to do it. Like a cough suppressant, or allergy medication.

- Don't lift ... well, almost anything really ... for at least the first 8 weeks. Longer if you're at high risk. Not a basket of laundry. Or a roast chicken. Or a baby. See the *Think Like a Survivalist* section in Chapter 1 for more information about what *not* to lift.

- Grocery shopping, for example, involves a surprising amount of lifting – lifting things off the shelves and into your cart, out of the cart at the cash, toting bags to the car, then into your home, then putting them away. Each small item or step might not seem significant, but it adds up. At the end of the day, you've done an awful lot of lifting and toting. Be extra cautious about this – smaller, more frequent trips to the store, enlisting help, whatever it takes.

- Go easy on chores like gardening, vacuuming, changing sheets, or anything that requires physical exertion. Wave a feather duster around if you must, but otherwise let these chores pile up or rely on others to do the dirty work for now.

- Getting up from a bed can strain the stomach muscles. Roll out of bed instead of sitting straight up. Or install a bed rail, like they have in hospitals but smaller.

- After about 8 weeks, you can supposedly start lifting and return to most normal activities again, within reason. But don't rush it. Check with your doctor to make sure you've healed well. Listen to your body and don't try to be a hero. Take a few months. If you're at high risk, take a year! There's no time limit on protecting yourself.

- A few months after ostomy surgery, you might want to consult a physiotherapist trained in techniques to gradually improve abdominal muscle tone, particularly in folks who've had surgery. If they tell you to do sit-ups or lift weights, then run *(away)!* But modified sit-ups with bent knees, pelvic tilts, swimming, walking, Pilates, etc. – these are all good.

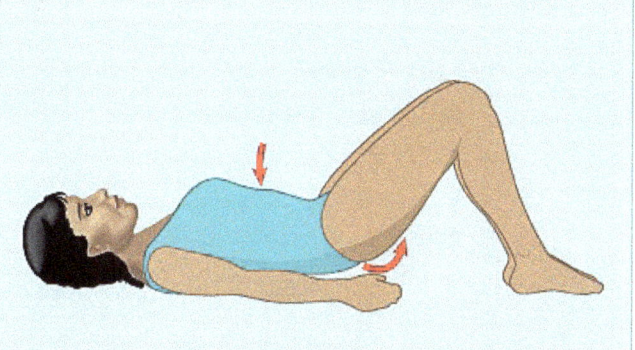

**Pelvic tilting**
1. Lie on your back on a firm surface with knees bent and feet flat on the bed
2. Pull your tummy in, tilt your bottom upwards slightly while pressing the middle of your back into the bed and hold for two seconds
3. Let go slowly

## Treatment of hernias

You've basically got two options – surgery or no surgery (at least for now). This isn't a time for home remedies. A squirt of baby oil or eating a few marshmallows aren't going to do the trick here. This is a decision you must make with your doctor.

WHAT COULD POSSIBLY GO WRONG?

## 1. Non-surgical

If the hernia is small and not causing any problems, your doctor might recommend a more conservative, management approach rather than surgery. At least for now. Hernia surgery has a pretty high recurrence rate. And the more surgeries you have, the higher the risk that it will happen again. So it's not something to be done in haste.

Here are some things you can do to try to avoid or delay surgery (if your doctor says you can wait):

- Wear a hernia belt, which is different from a hernia *prevention* belt. Make sure you're carefully measured for this. It isn't something to order off the shelf, like a support garment. Best to have a stoma nurse measure you and order it, if possible. There are many factors to consider, and several very specific measurements needed.

> *If your hernia belt bunches up painfully at the waist (more common in women, particularly those of us with "jelly bellies"), order a belt with extra stays across the back, not just at the sides. It may have to be custom-made, but if you can afford the extra expense, it's well worth it!*

- Most hernia belts are made with a hole for the pouch to come through. There *are* hernia belts with no holes. They're most common in Europe. The rationale for this type of belt is that putting a hole in the belt is basically recreating the situation that gave you the hernia in the first place – providing an opening for intestines to push through. Two stoma nurses have assured me that these belts don't cause pancaking. That may be because they don't hold your abdomen in as tightly as you might need if your hernia is pretty big. But if it's relatively small, you might want to try out a hernia belt with no hole.

- Put the hernia belt on before you get out of bed in the morning. If you have to take it off during the day, lie down for 5–10 minutes before putting it back on. This is to give your herniated intestines a chance to slip back inside as much as they can, which is where you want them to be when you put on the belt. If you allow the intestines to come out more, bulging out between your abdominal muscles and the skin surface, then all you're doing with the belt is squeezing them, which can lead to problems. Even if your hernia doesn't look like it reduces in size when you lie down, you can tell by pressing on it. After you've laid down for a while, it will probably feel softer.

- Be *extremely* careful about abdominal strain, as discussed above. At this point, you already have a hernia. It won't take much to make it grow larger. It may even grow larger on its own, but at least don't help it along.

- This is a good time to cut down on your risk factors for a recurrence, in case you do end up having the hernia repaired surgically somewhere down the road. You can't change some things, but you can try to lose weight if that's an issue, cut down on smoking, work on getting diabetes or blood pressure under control, that kind of thing.

## 2. Surgical

The following is general information about hernia repair surgery, to help you have an informed discussion with your doctor.

Speaking of doctors, be sure your surgeon is experienced in hernia repairs. Try to avoid a general surgeon who hasn't done a lot of them. Hernia repairs are typically the domain of colorectal surgeons or trauma surgeons. If you're fortunate enough to live near a hernia center, that could be a good option. Hernias are all they deal with. But even then, make sure the surgeon is experienced with parastomal hernias.

Don't hesitate to ask questions at your first consultation with a surgeon. For example, you might want to ask ...

- Why are you recommending surgery over non-surgical management of my hernia?
- Have you done many hernia repairs?
- What technique would you use (e.g., open or laproscopic?), and why?
- Will you use a mesh? Why or why not?
- Will you re-locate my stoma to another position on my abdomen? Why or why not?
- What are the risks in my particular case, including the risk of recurrence?
- Do you have any recommendations to reduce those risks?
- How long will I probably be in the hospital?
- What can I expect after surgery?
- Will the incision affect the placement or adhesion of my baseplate, short-term or long-term?
- Will I need any kind of home care?
- Am I likely to need a wound vac, JP drain, or negative pressure device (explained on next pages) during recovery?
- What are some normal symptoms I might experience during recovery, that I shouldn't worry about?
- What symptoms would warrant a call to you or a visit to ER?

Here's a little overview of hernia surgery, to help you understand the answers to some of those questions:

The surgery is either done laparoscopically (through a few tiny "keyhole" incisions) or "open" (a full incision in the abdomen).

A mesh is often used to reinforce the tissue surrounding the repair. This significantly reduces the chance of the hernia recurring. Although it carries a small risk of infection, it's generally the technique of choice and preferred over simply stitching up the opening in your abdominal wall after your intestines have been pushed back inside.

A parastomal hernia might be repaired and the stoma left where it is, or it might be repaired and your stoma moved to a new location on your abdomen.

After surgery, blood and other body fluids can build up inside, which can slow healing or cause infection. There are two ways to drain this fluid. Both types of drains may be left in place for varying lengths of time, from days to weeks, as determined by your doctor.

- With a wound vac, the wound is left open with a tube coming out, leading to a portable vacuum machine that "sucks the gunk out" while you're healing. The wound is covered with a dressing that's changed regularly, usually by in-home nurses.

- With a Jackson Pratt ("JP") drain, the surgical wound is closed, but you're left with a thin tube poking out, draining the fluids into a squeezable bulb attached at the end. You empty the bulb as needed, into the toilet. You may be asked to keep track of how much fluid accumulates in the bulb every day, what color it is, etc.

WHAT COULD POSSIBLY GO WRONG?

Negative pressure wound therapy (NPWT) is another option your surgeon might use to speed healing and reduce infection. After the incision is closed, a small vacuum device is placed over the wound. It literally sucks up debris and fluid on your skin, increases blood flow to the area, and all kinds of other good stuff. It can stay in place for several days or longer.

For tips on making life easier during your recovery from surgery, see the *Take Time to Heal* section of Chapter 2.

# FAQs
(Frequently Asked Questions)

---

## How often should I change my baseplate?

There's no one-size-fits-all answer to that question. It's different for each individual, and can even change from day to day for the same individual. It ranges from multiple times a day to once a week or even longer.

The best answer is to go as long as you can between changes, as long your skin is healthy and there are no leaks underneath.

Changing too often, like a few times a day, can damage the skin. And going too long between changes can increase the risk of something bad happening under there that you're not aware of (cue ominous music).

An online support group I belong to recently ran an informal survey of its members. About 75 responded (roughly half ileostomies, half colostomies). The average duration between changes was 4-5 days. Of course, this is very unscientific. But it sounds pretty reasonable as an average. And it's a nice, safe range – although it may seem unattainable to those with a high output ileostomy or with significant skin and leakage problems.

## Sometimes it feels like a bowel movement wants to come out "the old way." Is that normal?

Absolutely. It might be mucus, as described in the next question. But if not, even if there's nothing there to come out, your brain could still be signaling your body to pass a bowel movement the way it's always done. Eventually, this "phantom urge" will fade away. In the meantime, sitting on the toilet and even bearing down (a little) can often trick the brain into thinking it's done its job.

FAQs

## I still pass something through my rectum sometimes. What's up with that?

It's most likely mucus, which is usually clear or white-ish, and this is a normal thing. If it's bloody, yellowy-green, foul smelling, or painful, tell your doctor about it. But don't panic – this can often be easily treated.

Mucus is produced in the intestines, where it acts as a lubricant so stool can pass through easily. The mucus normally passes out of your body with the stool, through the rectum. Having an ostomy (whether ileostomy or colostomy, end or loop) means your stool is redirected out of your body somewhere before it reaches the rectum. Any part of your intestine that remains intact below that point keeps chugging along in blissful ignorance, producing mucus that isn't needed any more. (Kind of sad, really. Like a faithful dog waiting at the garden gate for a master who's never coming back. Sniff.)

If you still have a rectum, the mucus will want to come out there. So you might have a "bearing down" feeling from time to time, as if there's a bowel movement wanting to come out the old way. If so, you can sit on the toilet like you used to, and push down gently to encourage it to pass. This can happen anywhere from a few times a day to every few weeks. For some people, it never happens at all – the mucus just quietly seeps out, like a discharge.

It's not normally a problem, but sometimes the mucus can build up into a ball that's harder to pass. Glycerine suppositories, which you push into your rectum, can help dissolve the ball so it will pass easier.

I've also heard of folks who irrigate their rectum regularly to keep the mucus flowing. They use a small enema bottle or the kind of irrigation bulb that's used for babies' noses, filled with a little warm water and a few drops of aloe vera juice, glycerin soap, or distilled white vinegar. It just flushes the area out. Doesn't work for everyone but harmless, and worth a try.

If you experience more serious problems, like a blockage that prevents the mucus from coming out, your doctor may suggest a mucous fistula (like another stoma, only it's for mucous to come out, instead of stool).

## Why does my stoma have two holes?

When you have a loop ostomy, your intestine hasn't been completely severed. Instead, a loop of intestine was brought up to form the stoma, and a hole was made in it for your output to come out. There's usually a second hole made too, for mucus to come out from the part of the intestine below the stoma, because although no stool is going through there anymore, mucus is still being produced. That second hole is called the mucous fistula and is often so small that you may not even be aware of it.

## What's a Barbie butt?

It's a good-natured nickname for a female ostomate whose rectum has been removed and anus surgically closed. Barbie® dolls have no bum holes either. For the same reason, many male ostomates call themselves G.I. Joe butts, after the G.I. Joe® action figure. Other terms you may hear are "semi-colon" (someone who's had part of their colon removed) and "butt-crappers" (non-ostomates). Extra points if you can use that last one in conversation without a self-satisfied snicker.

## What can I do to control high output with an ileostomy?

When you first get an ileostomy, the output can be quite high, and then it settles into a routine - typically about 900 ml (3-4 cups) a day, or about 6 pouch changes. If the output suddenly increases, and this is unusual, it's probably regular old diarrhea. But if your level of output is always high, about 1500-2000 ml (6-8 cups) in 24 hours, or about 8-10 pouch changes or more a day, then it's considered "high output" or "ileostomy diarrhea."

This can cause problems like malnutrition, dehydration, electrolyte imbalance, and weight loss. And so much liquid output puts you at more risk for leaks.

The goal is to slow down the transit time of your food (to give your body more time to absorb the nutrients) and to thicken or bulk up your output to make it less watery. Here are some ways to do that:

# FAQs

- Eat frequent, small meals. Have a little something every couple of hours if you can. This helps your body absorb the nutrients.

- Include proteins and low fiber, starchy foods like potatoes, pasta, and bread, with every meal. These will slow down the transit time, giving your body more time to absorb the nutrients.

- Eat foods that thicken your output. See the *Food Charts* for diarrhea in Appendix A for a list of suggested foods that do this for many people.

- The output from ileostomies contains a large amount of sodium (salt). So with high output, you might become low in salt, as well as in potassium and other minerals and electrolytes. See the *Food Charts* for diarrhea for a list of recommended foods that are high in potassium.

Some ileostomates with high output wear high output drainable pouches at night that connect to a drainage bag, so they don't have to keep getting out of bed.

> Some people with a high level of watery output put a tampon in their pouch, to absorb liquid and cut down on sloshing. Very creative!

## What happens if I need a colonoscopy?

Most ostomates have had colonoscopies in the years before their surgeries, and it's natural to wonder how that will work now that they've got a stoma. There's no singular approach to the procedure in ostomates because there are so many variables (ileostomy/colostomy, end/loop, rectum/no rectum, presence/absence of medical issues like Crohn's disease, etc.). But here's an overview of the main elements:

# FAQs

No-one enjoys the prep for a colonoscopy, particularly drinking the purgative medication to clean and empty the bowel. But personally, I find it much easier with a colostomy. Instead of frequent mad dashes to the toilet with only seconds to spare, now when I feel another gusher coming, I calmly finish whatever I'm doing, let the pouch fill, and then stroll into the bathroom to empty it before the next round. No panic. No fuss, no muss. No burning rectum, like some non-ostomates have. All very civilized.

If you don't ordinarily use a drainable pouch, this is a good time to wear one. If you're worried about over-filling the pouch, particularly if you think it's going to continue overnight, you can switch to a bigger pouch. There are even "high output" drainable pouches, with a soft tap at the bottom that can be connected to a drainage bag. They're principally designed for ileostomates with high output, so they don't have to get out of bed several times during the night. If you've timed your colonoscopy prep so that you're pretty much emptied out by bedtime, this probably won't be necessary.

As far as the procedure itself is concerned, the tube may be inserted in your rectum, if you have one, just like before, and/or through your stoma. Remember there are no nerve endings in the stoma, so the insertion can actually be more comfortable this way. The overwhelming majority of ostomates who do this report little or no discomfort.

If it's through your stoma, you may be able to leave the baseplate on for the procedure and just remove the pouch. Either way, bring a full change with you just in case, and be prepared to reattach it yourself afterwards. The attending nurse may not be familiar with ostomies.

A word about virtual colonoscopies, also called CT-scan colonoscopies or CT colonographies. As the name suggests, this is a procedure where a CT-scan machine takes images of your colon from *outside* your body (rather than a camera at the end of a flexible tube inserted *into* your body). A thin catheter is inserted a tiny bit inside, through your rectum or stoma, to blow gas into your intestine to

# FAQs

make everything more visible (same as in a regular procedure). A thin balloon is inflated to prevent the catheter from slipping out or gas escaping. But that's all. The rest is images taken by a computer from outside your body. Virtual colonoscopies are generally considered to be at least as safe and accurate as regular ones, and much less invasive (so less risk of pain or discomfort, and less need for anesthetic, sedative, or pain relievers). Remember, though, that if anything suspicious is found, you'll still have to have a regular colonoscopy later, to treat it or to take a tissue sample for investigation.

## Is there a trick to using a 'click on' system? I'm hurting myself trying to push the pouch on!

First of all, if you're still recovering from surgery, this may not be the best time to use this type of 2-piece appliance - called a mechanical coupling. In the early days, you might be better off with an adhesive coupling that doesn't require pressing down hard on your abdomen.

But if you're well healed, a mechanical appliance can be a great choice. It just takes some getting used to.

If you're having trouble, apply a little water or liquid soap around the top of the flange with your finger. The flange is the protruding ring you're trying to click the pouch onto.

You can also try a low-pressure adapter. This is a device that goes between the baseplate and the pouch. Once attached to the flange, you can get your fingers underneath it - so you're attaching the pouch by squeezing your fingers together, not pressing against your abdomen.

They also make baseplates with "accordion flanges." Same idea. There's room for your fingers underneath the flange, making it easier to attach the pouch.

## Why can't I get the pouch to stay on when I use a bag liner with a 2-piece 'click & lock' system?

If you're having trouble, press the pouch (with the protruding bag liner) onto the flange and circle around it with your fingers, pressing firmly like you do normally (without a bag liner). But this time keep one hand there, maintaining that pressure and holding the pouch firmly in place against the flange. Use your other hand to squeeze the locking mechanism till it clicks. Then let go and give a gentle tug to make sure it's secure. You might have to try this a few times to get the hang of it, but it works. With a liner in it, the pouch will never hold on by itself. You need the lock to grab and hold it.

I find that a brand-new pouch can be hard to click onto a flange when there's a bag liner in there. But after it's been on for a while, it gets much easier to pop on and off. I eventually figured out it was because the hole in the pouch had stretched a little. Doh! So now I keep a supply of new pouches (with the liners inserted) clicked onto baseplates. It's much easier to attach them when they're not on your body. I leave them in my supply drawer until the next time I need a new pouch. At that point, I take one off a baseplate and voilà – a pre-stretched pouch!

## Why is my stool suddenly colored?

The first time you see any color in your stool, particularly red, it can be pretty scary. Don't panic.

Blackish stool can mean old blood, but it can also be a temporary result of eating dark chocolate or black licorice. Or it might be a harmless side effect of iron pills or transfusions, or PEPTO-BISMOL®, an OTC medication used to treat digestive upsets that's known to cause black stool in some folks (harmlessly).

If it's any other color of the rainbow, it's almost definitely something you ate. I've heard of people whose output turns bright neon green when they eat raspberry sherbet or drink a grape-flavored sports drink. Go figure!

# FAQs

Of course, if it's really blood in your stool, you should seek medical help. But take a few minutes first to think about what you've eaten recently that might explain why you're pooping in technicolor. Here are some common culprits:

- Beets
- Asparagus
- Spinach
- Tomato sauce
- Berries (red, black, or blue)
- Gelatin desserts like JELL-O®
- OREO® cookies or cereal
- Cough syrup
- Colored fruit punches or sports drinks
- Colored breakfast cereals
- Ice cream
- Licorice
- Red velvet cake
- Cotton candy
- Red wine

Remember that as always in ostomy world, different people have different reactions and experiences.

## Should I wear my hernia belt 24/7?

You don't need to, but you can if you feel more comfortable. Most people take hernia belts off for sleeping – and showering of course.

## What about sex?

This is a common area of concern for new ostomates. Bottom line: having an ostomy does not mean the end of a healthy, happy sex life. After surgery, check with your doctor when it's ok to resume that aspect of your life, or to risk pregnancy. But otherwise, you're good to go ... physically.

Mentally, that's a whole 'nother thing. Just like before your ostomy, self-image is an important factor in enjoying intimacy. If you feel bad about your body for any reason, it will affect both you and your partner. But if you're comfortable with yourself and accept that your ostomy is as much a part of you as wearing glasses, then the chances are that your partner will too.

Ostomates getting back into the dating world generally say that when they realize someone has potential, they bring up their ostomy after a few dates, before becoming intimate. This is uncharted territory for most folks you'll meet so they'll usually take their cue from you. If you present it as something you're comfortable with, they're likely to see it the same way. That's not to say there aren't a few jerks out there. But as some ostomates say, a stoma is a good "bullshit detector." The sooner you weed the jerks out, the sooner you can go onto bigger and better things.

I've heard countless stories of ostomates starting new physical relationships or resuming old ones, marrying, and having children. By far, the majority find that having an ostomy does not dampen their sex life, and in many cases even enhances it, as they discover new levels of openness, intimacy, and love.

This doesn't mean there are no boundaries at all. For those who practice anal sex, it's best to check with your doctor first because there may be restrictions based on what surgery you had and other medical factors. Some adventurous ostomates have wondered if they can have sex *in* their stomas. Now that's a definite no-no! It could do all kinds of damage to your stoma and intestines. And you probably wouldn't even be aware of it until it was too late, because there are no nerve endings in the stoma. It bears repeating: *Nothing* should ever be inserted into your stoma, except by a doctor. And even then only for medical reasons. If your sex partner happens to be a doctor, he doesn't get a free pass. LOL

Overall, the most common problem I've heard is that spouses and partners of ostomates can be afraid of intimacy at first. It's not that they don't want physical contact. They just have no idea how it feels and are afraid they're going to hurt you. If you can essentially say "Don't worry. I've got this!", it'll take a load off them. Show them that having an ostomy doesn't have to hold either of you back.

# FAQs

If you find it distracting to have a bag flapping around, you could wear a tummy support binder like a STEALTH BELT® that you can tuck your pouch into. You can put the pouch on horizontally under the binder. Or you could change to a smaller pouch, even a mini-pouch or stoma cap, if you're reasonably sure you won't have much output for a while. If you have any discomfort (e.g., because of the location of your stoma, or because of a hernia, etc.), find new positions that are more comfortable.

Basically, enjoying physical intimacy shouldn't be any more anxiety-producing after an ostomy than it was before.

## Sometimes I feel alone in the world. How many ostomates are out there?

Numbers are hard to come by, but according to most reliable resources, about 1 in 500 people in the western world have an ostomy. Thousands of new ostomates have their surgeries every year.

Most are colostomies, and most ostomies are permanent.

The most common causes of ostomies are colorectal cancer and IBD, including ulcerative colitis and Crohn's disease.

In practical terms, most of us never knew anyone with an ostomy before our surgeries – or thought we didn't – so it feels much rarer than it is. But if you mention having an ostomy in conversations, it's surprising how many other people will reveal they have one too, or know someone who does. That makes sense, if 1 in every 500 people in your community is an ostomate.

So the bottom line is this: There are ostomates all over the place. Most of them willing, even anxious, to share information and support with others – in books, in support groups, in person, online, wherever and however they can. You're not alone by any means! Just reach out and you'll find there's a world of support waiting for you.

# Epilogue

## THE OSTOMY RAFT

So we're all floating lazily down the river of life, each in our own boat ... when something goes terribly wrong. It could be a mechanical failure. Maybe your boat has sprung a slow leak. Or out of the blue you're attacked by pirates and tossed overboard. Whatever the reason, you find yourself alone in the water, arms flailing, desperately struggling to stay afloat.

Before too long an enormous raft appears in the distance. It's heading directly towards you. As it gets closer, you see it's filled with people. Just as you think it's about to run you over, all these strong arms and hands reach down from the raft and pull you to safety. Phew!

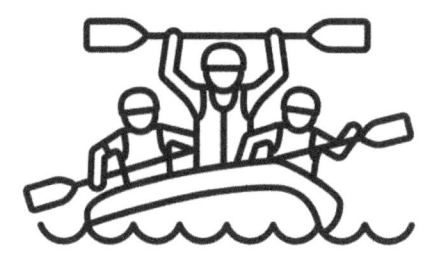

It takes a while to get your bearings. You're exhausted from your ordeal, maybe a little battered and bruised. But slowly, you begin to realize that everyone else on the raft is a survivor too. Some are still wet behind the ears. A few are only there temporarily, while their boats are being repaired. Others have been on the raft for years and know they'll be there for the rest of their journey. And that's ok.

Over time, you realize how lucky you are to be in such good company. You're still the same person, still floating down the same river. There's just been a change in your boat. And now you're ready to reach out and help others. After all, that's what the journey's all about.

# GLOSSARY

**Abdominoperineal resection (APR)** – Surgical procedure where the end of the colon, the rectum, and the anal sphincter are removed, resulting in a permanent colostomy.

**Adhesion** – Fibrous scar tissue, often from a surgery, that binds two surfaces together. In an ostomate, this could mean two sides of the intestine joining together at one spot, forming an obstruction.

**Adhesive remover** – A product can used to help remove a baseplate or any leftover adhesive on the skin after a baseplate's been removed. It comes in individual packets of wipes or as a spray.

**Adynamic obstruction** – *(see paralytic ileus)*

**Allergic dermatitis** – A type of contact dermatitis, where skin becomes red, sore, or irritated upon contact with a particular substance. Very similar to irritant dermatitis, but in this case, your skin is not simply irritated by the substance. This is an immune response. You're actually allergic to it. An allergy might not develop immediately, but only after the exposure is prolonged or repeated frequently. It can even take months to develop. Allergic dermatitis is more likely than irritant dermatitis to itch than to burn or sting, and more likely to form oozing blisters.

**Anastomosis** – Surgical procedure where two cut ends of intestine are rejoined. This is what happens when an end ostomy is reversed.

**Bag liner** – A transparent bag that's inserted into a pouch to collect output. To empty, the liner is simply pulled out of the pouch and discarded, leaving the pouch clean. A new liner is then inserted.

**Barrier** – *(see baseplate)*

# Glossary

**Barrier spray or wipe** – This is applied to form an invisible protective layer between your skin and the baseplate. It comes in a spray or in a wipe, which is daubed on. It's often used in crusting.

**Baseplate** – The baseplate (also known as a "barrier" or "wafer") is the part of the ostomy appliance that adheres to your abdomen, with a pouch attached. A hole in the baseplate allows your stoma to poke through.

**Bowel resection** – A surgical procedure where part of your small or large intestine is removed – *(see also colectomy and enterectomy)*

**Colectomy** – Surgical procedure where all or part of your colon (large intestine) is removed.

**Colon** – Another name for the large intestine.

**Colonoscopy** – Procedure where a long flexible tube, with a light and tiny camera attached, is inserted through the anus or through a stoma, into the large intestine, allowing the inside to be seen. A "virtual colonoscopy" is a CT-scan of your large intestine. In this case, there's no tube moving through your intestines, but only a small tube inserted just inside the anus or stoma to inflate the intestines with air, for a better image.

**Colostomate** – Someone who has a colostomy.

**Colostomy** – One end of your large intestine is brought out through a hole (or "stoma") in your abdomen, and creates a new way for stool to leave your body.

**Coupling ring** – *(see flange)*

**Crusting** – Many skin irritations are treated with powders. Because a baseplate won't adhere well to powder, a barrier wipe or spray is applied on top, to seal in the powder. Sometimes, you may need to apply 2-3 layers of powder & barrier product. This is called crusting.

**Digestive tract** – The muscular tract your food travels through, from when it goes in through your mouth to when it leaves your body through the anus (typically). It includes the small & large intestines.

**Double barrel stoma** – *(see mucous fistula)*

**Dynamic obstruction** – *(see mechanical blockage)*

**Electrolytes** – salts and minerals absorbed by the body, in the intestines.

**End ostomy** – Your intestine is cut and one end is brought up to your abdomen. The rest may be removed but is usually sewn shut and left inside your body. An end ostomy only has one hole, and is usually permanent (versus a loop ostomy, which has two holes and is usually temporary).

**Enterectomy** – A surgical procedure where part of the small or large intestine is removed.

**Enterostomal therapy nurse** – *(see stoma nurse)*

**Excoriation** – A breakdown of the skin. This can lead to an area around the stoma being weepy and/or bleeding.

**Extended wear baseplate** – resists moisture so it should last longer than a standard baseplate for people with ileostomies or loose stools.

**Fistula** – An opening, like a passageway, between two organs in the body, or between one organ and the skin. For example, a rectovaginal fistula is an opening between the rectum and vagina. Most fistulas happen as a result of some kind of trauma, like cancer, an abscess, radiation, etc. Others, like a mucous fistula, are created deliberately by a surgeon for medical reasons.

**Flange** – A rigid, protruding ring that circles the hole in a baseplate. In a 2-piece appliance, the pouch clicks or snaps onto the flange. Occasionally, people say "flange" when they're referring to a baseplate.

# Glossary

**Flange extenders** – Optional adhesive strips that you apply around the edges of your baseplate to make it extra secure. They're usually C-shaped or Y-shaped. It's actually a misnomer. They're really "baseplate extenders."

**Floating flange** – The flange on the baseplate is raised a little so you can slip a thumb or finger under it to help click on the pouch.

**Gastrointestinal (GI) tract** – *(see digestive tract)*

**Granuloma** – A small, red bump of tissue around the peristomal area (on or around the stoma). Granulomas often appear in clusters and often around the edge of the stoma, where it meets the skin. They may cause no problem, or may bleed easily and be uncomfortable.

**Hernia** – A bulge created when an organ pushes through the muscle or tissue that contains it. For ostomates, this is usually when some of your intestine push out through the passageway made for your stoma. The intestines form a bulge within the abdominal cavity. This can also happen after a stoma has been closed, and the incision in your abdominal muscle re-opens.

**Hernia belt** – A belt worn by people with hernias. There are many sizes, types, and fabrics to choose from. It's worn over the baseplate and generally has a hole for the pouch to stick out through, so you may be able to empty the pouch without removing the belt. You need to be carefully measured for a hernia belt, to ensure it will fit your ostomy appliance exactly. It should be worn all day, every day, not just when you're going to be lifting something.

**Ileoanal reservoir/ileoanal pouch** – *(see J-pouch)*

**Ileostomate** – Someone who has an ileostomy.

**Ileostomy** – One end of your small intestine is brought out through a hole (or "stoma") in your abdomen, and creates a new way for your waste (mostly liquid at this point) to leave the body.

**Ileus** – *(see paralytic ileus)*

# Glossary

**Inflammatory Bowel Disease (AKA Irritable Bowel Disorder) (IBD)** - A long-term inflammation of the digestive tract. There are different forms of IBD, mainly Crohn's disease and ulcerative colitis. IBD is different from Irritable Bowel Syndrome (IBS), which does not cause inflammation or damage to the GI tract.

**Irrigation** - A way for colostomates to manage their bowel movements, training them to happen on a schedule. It's basically a water enema that flushes out the stool in the large intestine. Irrigation takes about an hour, and is done daily by some colostomates and a few times a week by others. The idea is that after evacuating its contents, the large intestine will take a day or two to refill. In the meantime, you can wear a simpler appliance, like a stoma cap or a mini-pouch, and probably won't need to empty it very often, or even at all, between irrigations.

**Irritant dermatitis** - A type of contact dermatitis, where skin becomes red, sore, or irritated upon contact with a particular substance, including feces. It often looks like a burn. Very similar to allergic dermatitis, but in this case, you're not actually allergic to the substance. Instead, your skin just reacts to it severely, and usually more quickly than an allergic reaction - often with the first exposure. Irritant dermatitis is more likely than allergic dermatitis to burn or sting, and the irritated skin is more likely to look swollen.

**J-Pouch** - (also known as an "ileoanal reservoir" or "ileoanal pouch"). This is an internal, J-shaped reservoir for stool made from a loop of your small intestine. It's brought down to the anus and a hole is made in the pouch for the stool to pass out of your body. This is done in patients whose large intestine and rectum have been removed. The sphincter muscle remains intact, so once the J-pouch is healed and functioning, the stool passes out through your anus as it always did, and you still have the muscle control to hold it in when necessary. While it heals, you'll probably have a temporary ileostomy.

**Jackson Pratt (or "JP") drain** - A method of draining out fluids that can build up inside the body and cause infection or slow down healing after a surgery. The wound is closed, but a narrow tube is left in place and pokes through a small opening in the skin. Fluid drains through the tube into a bulb at the end. You

# Glossary

empty the bulb into the toilet as needed. When the draining slows down, as determined by the doctor, the tube is pulled out.

**Laparoscopic surgery** – A surgery that's performed not with a large, open incision, but by inserting implements including a camera through a few small incisions.

**Large intestine** – After food has made its way through your small intestine, where most of the nutrients were absorbed, it moves into your large intestine – which is about 5 feet or 1½ meters long. It's mostly liquid at first. But as it moves through the large intestine, the water (along with electrolytes and other nutrients and vitamins) are absorbed into your body. Whatever's left over is "bulked up" to form stool. Waves of muscle contractions in the large intestine move the stool along till it reaches the rectum (typically) and leaves your body. In a colostomate, the stool exits your body through your stoma at some point in the large intestine before it reaches the rectum.

**Loop ostomy** – A loop of your intestines is brought up to the surface of your tummy and two holes are made in the intestine. Stool or output passes through one hole, and small amounts of mucus come out the other. A loop ostomy is usually temporary.

**Low-pressure adapter** – A device, like a coupling ring, that goes between the baseplate and the pouch to make it easier to press the pouch onto the baseplate. It's often used in the post-surgery period, when the abdomen is tender and pressure on it might be painful.

**Lubricating deodorant** – An optional product that's squirted into a pouch or bag liner to encourage the stool to drop down and not collect around the stoma. It also includes a deodorant to reduce or mask smells.

**Lumen** – The internal channel of your intestine, through which the stool passes, ending in an opening in your stoma.

# Glossary

**Mechanical blockage** – (also known as "dynamic obstruction"). This is a physical obstruction in the intestine, caused by a build-up of food or by a structural blockage, like an adhesion from scar tissue.

**Mechanical coupling** – This refers to how the pouch attaches to the baseplate on a 2-piece appliance. The baseplate has a protruding ring (the flange) that the pouch presses or clicks onto in a variety of ways, depending on the brand and style.

**Mucocutaneous separation**– This is when the stoma separates from the skin around it. This can happen for a few reasons, including poor wound healing due to malnutrition, diabetes, radiation, etc., and is susceptible to infection, like any open wound.

**Mucous fistula** – An opening for mucus. Mucus is secreted in the intestines and acts as a lubricant. It normally passes out of your body with regular stool. Mucous fistulas can appear in different ways:

With a loop ostomy, two holes are usually created in the stoma – one for stool and one for mucus. You may not see the small mucus hole. Many people with loop ostomies don't even know it exists. Output from both holes (feces and mucus) collects in the one ostomy pouch.

With an end ostomy, occasionally both ends of the intestine are brought to the surface of your skin as two separate stomas – one for feces or stool, and one for mucus (the mucous fistula). This is called a "double barrel stoma." Everything above the stoma passes out the first hole, like any ostomy. Whatever portion of your intestines is left below the stoma is only producing mucous now – which normally passes out of your body through the rectum. But if there's a problem there (like a blockage), a second stoma might be required for the mucous to pass through (the mucous fistula). The two stomas may be close together or on two different places on your abdomen. A separate mucous fistula doesn't need a whole ostomy appliance, but a small one like a stoma cap may do the job, or even just a dressing to cover it.

# Glossary

**Necrosis** – Necrosis of the stoma means the blood supply to or from the stoma has been restricted or cut off. The stoma will likely turn a dark color. If so, this requires immediate medical attention.

**Negative pressure wound therapy (NPWT)** – A small vacuum device placed on top of a closed incision after surgery to speed healing and reduce infection.

**Ostomy** – An opening in the intestines or urinary system, through which body fluids such as waste or urine passes out of the body and is collected in a pouch. Colostomies, ileostomies, and urostomies are all different types of ostomies.

**Ostomy reversal** – *(see anastomosis)*

**Pancaking** – When stool doesn't drop down into the pouch, but builds up around the stoma. It's often a mushy consistency.

**Paralytic ileus** – (also known as "adynamic obstruction" or "ileus"). This happens when the normal muscle contractions in the intestine stop, so the contents of your bowels don't move.

**Parastomal hernia** – A hernia formed in the area of your stoma. It usually appears as a round bulge under the stoma. It can be quite small or very big.

**Paste** – A putty-like product that comes in a tube or strip. It's used to fill in gaps or dents in the skin, to create an even surface for the baseplate to stick to.

**Peristalsis** – A series of muscle contractions, like waves, that move contents like food and stool through the digestive system, including through the intestines.

**Peristomal skin** – The skin around your stoma, usually covered by the baseplate.

**Pouch** – Most ostomates simply refer to this as a "bag." It's the pouch that attaches to the baseplate and collects the stool.

**Proctectomy** – Surgical procedure where all or part of the rectum is removed.

**Proctocolectomy** – Surgical procedure where the rectum and all or part of the colon (large intestine) is removed.

## Glossary

**Prolapsed stoma** – A stoma normally protrudes about 2 cm or ¾" out of your abdomen. If it's pushed out much more than that (sometimes up to 10 cm or 4" or even longer), it's called prolapsed. This is more common in colostomies than ileostomies, and especially in loop colostomies. A prolapsed stoma is somewhat like a hernia and like a hernia, it can be managed conservatively or repaired with surgery.

**Pyroderma gangrenosum** – A ulcer, like an open sore. It can be anywhere on your body and isn't limited to people with ostomies, but those with GI diseases like ulcerative colitis or Crohns disease have increased risk so it's a known complication of ostomies (usually appearing beside the stoma).

**Rectal stump** – The portion of your intestines that's left below the stoma (i.e., between your stoma and your rectum) with an end ileostomy or end colostomy. It's no longer attached to your digestive system so there's no stool passing through it, just mucous being secreted. If your rectum has been removed, you don't have a rectal stump. The rectum and any intestines below the stoma are gone.

**Rectum** – The lowest part of your large intestine, just above the anus. Stool is stored here until it's passed out of your body.

**Retracted stoma** – The opposite of a prolapsed stoma. When the stoma is flush with the skin or below the skin level, it's called retracted. It's more common with ileostomies than colostomies, and more common in people who are heavier. The main problem associated with retracted stoma is leaking or pancaking, because the stoma doesn't stick out enough to drop output into the pouch. Instead, it often tends to seep under the baseplate or collect around the stoma opening.

**Revision** – A surgery to reconstruct an existing stoma or to close the existing stoma and relocate it to a different place on your abdomen.

**Short bowel syndrome** – (also called "short gut"). A condition where all or part of the small intestine has been removed or isn't functioning due to some disease

# Glossary

process. The most common complication is malnutrition, because most nutrients from our food are absorbed in the small intestine. A person with short bowel syndrome often relies on nutritional supplements.

**Small intestine** – After food is broken down in your stomach, it passes through the top half of your intestines (the small intestine, which is about 20 feet or 6 meters long). This is where most of the nutrients are absorbed. At this stage, it's mostly liquid. From there, it goes to the large intestine (typically) to be formed into stool before leaving your body. In ileostomates, this liquid or semi-liquid exits your body before it ever reaches the large intestine.

**Sphincter** – A circle-shaped muscle that surrounds an opening and allows you to control (close) it. The anus has a sphincter muscle. A stoma does not.

**Standard wear baseplate** – absorbs perspiration under the baseplate and provides good adhesion to the skin. Best for colostomies. Doesn't last as long as extended wear baseplates for people with loose, watery stool.

**Stenosis** – A narrowing of the internal channel of the intestine, through which the stool passes.

**Stoma** – Technically, a stoma is an opening in your body. But almost always, when an ostomate says "stoma," they mean the part of the intestine that's sticking out of their abdomen.

**Stoma bridge** – A product consisting of foam-like cubes that you stick inside your pouch to keep the two sides apart. It's designed to prevent pancaking.

**Stoma cap** – A small pouch that doesn't hold very much output but is frequently used for short periods when you might not want a larger appliance stuck to your abdomen (such as during intimacy, or under a swimsuit). It's also often worn by colostomates who irrigate, because their bowel movements are usually scheduled and predictable.

**Stoma collar** – A device that goes under the baseplate. A cylindrical "spout" protrudes through the hole in the baseplate, allowing the output to drop into the pouch. Used to prevent leaks.

**Stoma guard** – A rigid protector of the stoma, usually made of hard plastic. Good for protection from impact (like sports or jumping enthusiastic dogs), and anything that might constrict or press on the pouch and stoma (like seat belts and tight clothing).

**Stoma nurse** – Stoma nurses are certified specialists in the care of stomas and the support of ostomates. They work with pre-op and post-op patients, teach them how to manage their ostomies and how to treat problems. They're up-to-date on the latest ostomy products and can help you choose the best appliance and accessories for your particular needs.

**Transit time** – How long it takes food to go through your digestive system (i.e. in through the mouth and out through the stoma). For most people it's several hours, but it can vary widely.

**Wafer** – *(see baseplate)*

**Wound care nurse** – *(see stoma nurse)*

**Wound vac** – A therapy for wounds. After surgery, the wound is left open. A sponge is placed in it, as well as a draining tube. The opening is covered by a transparent membrane that sticks to the healthy skin around the wound, with the tube protruding out. Periodically, the tube is connected to a vacuum device that draws body fluid out. The dressing (including the sponge and transparent membrane) is changed periodically, usually by an in-home nurse. Wound vac therapy is done to promote faster healing and reduce infection in acute or chronic wounds.

# Appendix A

## FOOD TABLES

The following tables show a selection of foods and drinks to consume and those to avoid, to manage digestive problems that ostomates can run into.

If you have a condition like food allergies, diabetes, gluten intolerance, etc., you'll have to factor that into your selections. Hopefully, there are enough choices that you can find the right foods for your own unique needs.

**Note: These charts do NOT take into account other medical conditions (like IBD, diverticulitis, Celiac disease, etc.) that might have very different and specific dietary requirements.**

**If you have any kind of underlying disease or disorder always check with your doctor or registered dietician before making significant changes to your diet.**

APPENDIX A

# Gas

Passing gas is a natural process, but it can be particularly annoying or troublesome for ostomates. Here are some dietary tips to help reduce the build-up of excess gas in your body. (See the *Gas* section, Chapter 7, for more tips).

| | GAS | |
|---|---|---|
| | 👍 | 👎 |
| **BEVERAGES** | **Green juices** – Make juices or smoothies with kale, spinach or other green leafy vegetable. | **Carbonated or sparkling drinks** |
| | **Chamomile tea** – Best if brewed strong. | |
| | **Warm lemon water** – Squeeze the juice of a lemon into a glass of water. | **Alcoholic beverages** |
| **FRUIT** | **Berries** (strawberries, raspberries, blueberries, etc.) – Berries don't actively reduce gas, but they're low in sorbitol (which causes gas), so they're a good choice. | **Apples, bananas, cherries, citrus fruits, peaches, prunes, pears, raisins** – Many of these fruits contain a sugar called sorbitol. Citrus fruits have high levels of soluble fiber. Both can cause excess gas. |
| | **Papaya, pineapple** – Papaya and pineapple contain enzymes that break down food faster, creating less gas. | |

| | GAS, cont'd | |
|---|---|---|
| | 👍 | 👎 |
| **VEGETABLES** | **Pumpkin** – in any form | **Asparagus, broccoli, brussels sprouts, carrots, cauliflower, corn, cucumber, onions, radishes, sauerkraut, turnips/rutabaga** – Many of these vegetables contain types of sugars that cause gas when they're digested. |
| | **Fennel** – slice thin and add to salads or slaw | |
| | **Cabbage** – Despite its bad reputation, cabbage actually contains good bacteria that help break down foods so gas doesn't build up. | |
| | | **Potatoes** – starchy and high in carbohydrates, which can cause gas |
| **DAIRY** | **Probiotic yogurt, aged hard cheese, butter, sherbet** – These are lower in lactose (which can cause gas). | **Milk, ice cream, sour cream, puddings.** – Dairy products contain lactose, a sugar that can be difficult to digest and can cause gas – especially if you're lactose intolerant. |
| **LEGUMES** | | **Beans or peas, any soy product** – Beans contain a sugar found in vegetables on the "don't eat" list for gas, as well as soluble fiber. A double whammy! |

APPENDIX A

| | GAS, cont'd | |
|---|---|---|
| | 👍 | 👎 |
| **NUTS** | | Any nuts |
| **GRAINS** | **White rice** – Rice doesn't reduce gas, but unlike other starchy foods, it doesn't create gas either. So it's allowed. | **Oats (oat bran, oatmeal)** – Foods with high soluble fiber can cause gas. Oats are particularly high in this.<br><br>**Bread, pasta, etc.** – Starchy foods (except white rice) are high in carbohydrates, which can cause gas. |
| **FATTY FOODS** | | Fatty meats<br><br>Fried foods, including French fries<br><br>Rich sauces & gravies |

|  | GAS, cont'd | |
|---|---|---|
|  | 👍 | 👎 |
| **HERBS & SPICES** | **Peppermint** – Chew a few leaves raw or add them to tea | |
| | **Ginger** – Make gingerroot tea (pour boiling water over a chunk of ginger, add honey and lemon), or grate/purée ginger to add to soups. | |
| | **Basil, black pepper, cardamom, cayenne pepper, coriander, dill, marjoram, oregano, parsley, rosemary, cloves, savory, tarragon** – All these herbs are "carminative" – which means they prevent or reduce gas | |
| | **Dandelion greens** – sautéed or added to a salad | |
| **SUGARS** | **Raw honey** – about a spoonful | **Chocolate bars, candy, cookies, pastries, etc.** – any foods with a lot of sugar, which is a carbohydrate and can therefore cause gas. |

APPENDIX A

# Constipation

**Colostomates** – This chart shows some food & drinks to consume (or avoid) to help prevent or reduce constipation. (For more tips, see the *Constipation* section, Chapter 7).

 If your constipation becomes chronic, lasts unusually long, or causes pain, nausea, or vomiting, seek medical treatment.

**Ileostomates** – **This chart is NOT for you!** People with ileostomies rarely, if ever, suffer from constipation. A lack of output is far more likely to be blockage, which could actually be aggravated by following these recommendations.

| | CONSTIPATION | |
|---|---|---|
| | 👍 | 👎 |
| **BEVERAGES** | **Water** – Very important! | **Milk shakes** – A triple threat (dairy, high fat, sugary). |
| | **Hot drinks** – Especially coffee (in moderation) | |
| | **Juice** - Especially prune and pineapple juice. Juice with pulp contains more fiber. Some people say a glass of red grape juice makes them poop. Pear juice and apple juice are great if juiced with skins on. | |

| | CONSTIPATION, cont'd | |
|---|---|---|
| | 👍 | 👎 |
| **DAIRY** | | **Cheese, high fat milk, ice cream, sour cream, yogurt (regular, non-probiotic)** – Contain lactose, which can cause gas and worsen constipation |
| **FRUIT** | **Apples, apricots, avocados, berries, cherries, dates, dried fruit (prunes, raisins, figs, apricots), kiwis, oranges, papayas, peaches, pears, plums** – Most of these fruits contain high fiber. Many have other elements that relieve constipation and act as a natural laxative. Most of the fiber in apples & pears is in the skin – so organic is best, or at least wash the fruit well. Some (like cherries, peaches, apricots, & plums/prunes) work so well that eating too many will actually trigger diarrhea. So pace yourself. | **Unripe bananas** – Contain high levels of starch, which can worsen symptoms of constipation |

APPENDIX A

| | 👍 | 👎 |
|---|---|---|
| **CONSTIPATION, cont'd** | | |
| **VEGETABLES** | **Arugula, beets, broccoli, brussels sprouts, okra, cabbage, raw carrots, kale, legumes, turnips, spinach, sweet potatoes** – Most are rich in fiber, and many have other benefits for constipation. Beets have betacyanin, which helps fight cancer (especially colon cancer). Cook the green leafy tops like spinach. Cabbage is considered a natural laxative. Okra lubricates the intestinal tract, making it easier for stool to pass. | **Cooked carrots** – Some say cooking carrots can aggravate constipation. |
| **LEGUMES** | **Legumes** (peas, lentils & beans, including green beans) have more fiber than almost any other food. | |

| | CONSTIPATION, cont'd | |
|---|---|---|
| | 👍 | 👎 |
| PROTEINS | **Fish/Seafood** – Fish like salmon, tuna, mackerel, and halibut are a good source of magnesium, which helps draw water into your stool and make it easier to pass. Mollusks (like clams, mussels, scallops, oysters, and octopuses) are also high in magnesium. | **Red meats** – Contain large amounts of fat that slow down the digestive process, and protein fibers that are difficult to digest.<br><br>**Processed meats** – Hard to digest and contain nitrates, which can increase constipation. |
| GRAINS | **100% whole grain breads and cereals, brown rice** – Whole grain rye bread is particularly good for relieving constipation. | **Processed grains like white bread and white rice** – Low in fiber, can cause constipation |
| NUTS | **Chestnuts, almonds, pine nuts, pistachios, hazelnuts, peanuts, pecans** – all nuts are good sources of fiber. These ones are particularly good. | |

APPENDIX A

| | CONSTIPATION, cont'd | |
|---|---|---|
| | 👍 | 👎 |
| **SEEDS** | **Flaxseed, hemp seeds, sunflower seeds** – A good source of fiber. Sprinkle a tablespoon on smoothies, salads, or oatmeal. | |
| **SUGARS** | **Dark chocolate (70% cacao)** – A reasonably good source of magnesium. If you're craving something sweet, this is a good choice. | **Milk chocolate, cakes, pastries, doughnuts, etc.** – Low fiber/high fat combination can slow down the digestive symptom. |
| **FATTY FOODS** | | **Any fried foods, including French fries** – Hard to digest and high in fat, slowing down the digestive process. |
| **FROZEN DINNERS** | | **Most frozen dinners** – Typically low fiber/high fat. |

172

# Food blockages

**Ileostomates** – Try these tips if you're having normal output (what's normal for you) and want to prevent developing a food blockage. However, if you're having very reduced or watery output only, stop eating food entirely until it's resolved. And if you have no output at all, don't eat or drink anything. (For more tips, see the *Blockages* section, Chapter 7).

 If blockage symptoms aren't relieved in a reasonable amount of time, or you're in severe pain or vomiting – get to the ER!

**Colostomates** – Do NOT follow these recommendations, as you should be on a high fiber diet – which is pretty much the opposite of this regimen. If you're having reduced output, or none at all, it's far more likely to be constipation. However, if you believe you really are experiencing a blockage, follow the medical advice above (temporarily).

| | FOOD BLOCKAGES | |
|---|---|---|
| | 👍 | 👎 |
| **BEVERAGES** | **Water** – very important!! | **Smoothies** – with pulp or fiber |
| | **Juice** – Fruit and vegetable juices without pulp | **Juice** – Fruit and vegetable juices <u>with</u> pulp |

APPENDIX A

| | FOOD BLOCKAGES, cont'd. | |
|---|---|---|
| | 👍 | 👎 |
| **FRUIT** | Melons, apples (peeled & cooked), canned fruits (peaches, pears, apricots, etc.) | Oranges & grapefruits, grapes, pineapple, coconut, berries, dried fruit – Generally, avoid fruits with skins, pith, or seeds. |
| **VEGETABLES** | Squash, turnips, pumpkin, carrots (cooked), potatoes (without skin), tomato sauce & paste (no seeds), cucumbers (no seeds or skin), lettuce (shredded), zucchini (without skin). Cooked vegetables are better than raw, and shredded are better than large pieces. | Cabbage (raw), celery, corn, mushrooms, onions, spinach, Swiss chard, Chinese vegetables (bamboo shoots, water chestnuts) – Generally, avoid leafy greens, raw vegetables, and those with stalks, pips, or skin. |
| **LEGUMES** | | **Legumes** (peas, beans, lentils) are loaded with fiber, so avoid them entirely. |

Food Tables

| | 👍 | 👎 |
|---|---|---|
| **FOOD BLOCKAGES, cont'd.** | | |
| **DAIRY** | **Milk products**, including milk, pudding, creamy soups, and mild cheeses | **Yogurt containing fruit with seeds or skins** – like berries or cherries |
| **PROTEINS** | Egg, chicken, fish, meat (without gristle or connective tissue) | Meat (like steak) with gristle or connective tissue |
| | Peanut butter (smooth) | Peanut butter (crunchy) |
| **GRAINS** | **Refined flours** – White bread, pasta, rice, crackers, tapioca, processed cereals that aren't whole grain | **Whole grain products** – Multigrain or whole wheat bread, brown rice, whole grain pasta, muesli, etc. |
| **SNACKS** | | Nuts & seeds, popcorn, trail mix, granola, nutrition bars with fiber/grains |

APPENDIX A

# Diarrhea

Both ileostomates and colostomates can develop diarrhea. Follow these recommendations to help thicken your stool and to replenish electrolytes if you've lost a lot of liquid.

(For more tips, see the *Diarrhea* section, Chapter 7).

| | DIARRHEA | |
|---|---|---|
| | 👍 | 👎 |
| **BEVERAGES** | Tomato juice or V8® vegetable juice, carrot juice, orange or grapefruit juice, white grape juice, sports drinks (like GATORADE®), soups (*NOT* low-sodium) – liquids that replenish salt and/or potassium | Alcohol, caffeine, milk, most fruit juices (especially apple, prune, and red grape juice) – because they contain sorbitol, unlike citrus juices and white grape juice. Sorbitol can cause or aggravate diarrhea. |
| **FRUIT** | Bananas, applesauce – help to thicken stool | Prunes, dates, berries, pineapple, rhubarb, pears, melons |
| | Dried fruit, apricots, bananas, avocado, tomatoes/tomato sauce – to replenish potassium | |

# Food Tables

| | DIARRHEA, cont'd | |
|---|---|---|
| | 👍 | 👎 |
| **VEGETABLES** | Beets, butternut squash, Swiss chard, leafy greens – to replenish potassium | Cabbage, cauliflower, Brussels sprouts, corn |
| | Potatoes (without skin), including sweet potatoes – to thicken stool and replenish potassium | |
| **LEGUMES** | | **Legumes** (peas, beans, lentils) contain a lot of fiber, which can make diarrhea worse. |
| **DAIRY** | Probiotic yogurt & kefir | **Most other dairy products** – like milk, butter, ice cream, cheese, etc. |
| | **Dairy products with low lactose** – some people experience temporary lactose intolerance when they have diarrhea | |
| **PROTEINS** | Lean fish, beef, and pork. Skinless chicken | **Processed meats** – can contain too many fats and oils |
| | Peanut butter (smooth) | |

APPENDIX A

| | DIARRHEA, cont'd | |
|---|---|---|
| | 👍 | 👎 |
| GRAINS | Refined grains (like **white rice, bread, and pasta**), and grains with soluble fiber (like **oatmeal and cream of wheat** … but add these slowly). | Grains with insoluble fiber, like **whole wheat, bran products, wheat germ, whole grain bread, brown or wild rice** |
| SUGARS | | Honey, chocolate, licorice, artificial sweeteners |
| FATTY FOODS | | Fried or greasy foods, gravy |
| SNACKS | **Pretzels** – to replenish salt and/or potassium | **Nuts, pickles or olives**<br><br>**Gum** – too much can cause or aggravate diarrhea because most are sweetened with sorbitol – a natural laxative |

# Appendix B

# SYMPTOMS CHECKLIST

---

 *Important note:* The following chart contains descriptions of many of the most common symptoms associated with many of the most common complications in bowel ostomies. It's not an exhaustive list, by any means. Its sole purpose is to inform, and maybe help you describe what's happening to a medical professional. It's NOT intended to be used as a diagnostic tool or to replace medical advice. **In almost every case, these symptoms should be checked out by a stoma nurse, your family physician, or your surgeon.**

# APPENDIX B

| Category | Symptoms | Possible causes |
|---|---|---|
| BLEEDING | Mild, occasional, stops easily | Usually from a **mild trauma**, which might even be from wiping it while cleaning around the stoma. The stoma is full of blood vessels close to the surface, so it doesn't take much for it to bleed a little and this is normal. Could also be a small cut from the edge of the hole in the baseplate if the hole is too small or was cut a little ragged, or if the hole is too big and rubs around the stoma area. |
| | Bleeding from the hole (lumen) in the stoma | Often associated with an **underlying disease**, like Crohn's disease, among other causes. |
| | Bleeding from around the stoma | Could be **mucocutaneous separation**, where the stoma separates from the tissue around it. |
| | Bleeding from tiny bumps around the stoma | Might be **granulomas**. |
| RECTAL DISCHARGE | Clear or white, no smell | This is **normal** for ostomates who still have a rectum after surgery. It's a mixture of mucus and dead cells from the lining of the rectum and the part of your colon below the ostomy. |
| | Yellowish or green, strong smell, possibly traces of blood | This might be a sign of **infection**. |

## Symptoms Checklist

| Category | Symptoms | Possible causes |
|---|---|---|
| **SKIN PROBLEMS** | Red, itchy, shiny flat patches, with small raised white bumps | May be a **yeast or fungal infection** (candidiasis). The bumps might look like blisters. The skin might look puffy and there could be oozing. |
| | Wet, bumpy | Might be a "**mechanical irritation**," usually caused by removing the baseplate too frequently or washing the area too harshly. |
| | Pale or white, moist, wrinkly | Usually a sign of **prolonged exposure to moisture** under the baseplate. The skin softens and swells, and is easier to damage ("maceration"). Can lead to leaking. Often caused by excessive perspiration or applying the baseplate before the skin is completely dry. |
| | Burning or itchy, red rash, may be weepy. | Could be **contact dermatitis** – a reaction from exposure to feces or to a substance in a product (adhesive on baseplate, tape, soap, skin barriers, pouch material, etc.). The irritation can progress to blisters or welts.<br>• *Allergic contact dermatitis* is more likely to itch and to form blisters<br>• *Irritant contact dermatitis* is more likely to burn or sting, and to appear weepy. |

# APPENDIX B

| Category | Symptoms | Possible causes |
|---|---|---|
| **SKIN PROBLEMS, cont'd.** | Whitish, scaly patches | Often a sign of **psoriasis**, which can develop under the baseplate. May also be present on other parts of the body. |
| | Tiny, red, painful bumps | Might be an inflammation of hair follicles under the baseplate ("**folliculitis**"). Red pinpoints may appear at the base of the hair follicles. This can happen if you remove the hair around your stoma too often, or pull off the baseplate too forcefully. |
| | | Could also be **granulomas** – small nodules of tissue that may be on the stoma but are more often around it, next to the skin. They might bleed easily. They're harmless by themselves and can be painless, but can require treatment if they become uncomfortable or too large. |
| | Painful sores | May be **pressure ulcers**, caused by excessive pressure on the skin around the stoma – often from using convex baseplates. |
| | Painful open sores, irregularly shaped, look infected, with red or purple "rolled" or ragged edges | Can be **pyoderma gangrenosum**, a skin disease often associated with IBD. |

# Symptoms Checklist

| Category | Symptoms | Possible causes |
|---|---|---|
| **STOMA CHANGES** | Swelling | Stomas are typically swollen immediately **after surgery**, and gradually decrease in size over the next 6–8 weeks. But if you're not in the post-surgery period and it suddenly swells, there are a number of possible causes: |
| | | **Pre-bowel movements** – Some people's stomas swell just before a bowel movement, particularly if it's not coming out easily. After the bowel movement, the stoma returns to normal. |
| | | **Constipation** – particularly in colostomies. May be accompanied by symptoms such as little or no output, cramping, and/or nausea. |
| | | **Blockage** – particularly in ileostomies. May be accompanied by symptoms such as little or no output, a feeling of stomach churning, cramps, sweating, nausea, and/or vomiting. |
| | | **Prolapse** – a prolapsed stoma (one that's sticking out too far) often swells with fluid accumulation (edema). |
| | Movement in/out | The stoma might move in and out as you change positions. This is normal. If it's too excessive (i.e., if it "telescopes" too far out, or pulls back too far inside), this could be a prolapse or retraction. |

# APPENDIX B

| Category | Symptoms | Possible causes |
|---|---|---|
| STOMA CHANGES, cont'd. | Change in color | A **darkening** of the stoma, going from a moist, shiny red to a dark color (dark red, dusty blue/purple, brown, black) is usually a sign that the blood flow to and from your stoma has been compromised ("ischemia") and the tissue may be dying ("necrosis"). The stoma might also have a foul odor, and some of the tissue might slough off. |
| | | A stoma that changes to a **very pale** color is another sign of restricted blood flow and/or low hemoglobin and hematocrit levels, iron deficiency, etc. |
| | White or yellow streaks | Can be a sign of a **small cut or tear**, which is usually caused by the stoma rubbing against part of the baseplate. It may or may not bleed. |
| | Small white or pale yellow patches | Might be **ischemic ulcers**, caused by poor blood supply. May be seen more often in a prolapsed stoma. |
| | Burning/stinging | Burning or stinging inside the stoma while output is passing through it may be a reaction to eating spicy foods, like jalapenos, or a warning sign of **stenosis** (see next page). |

Symptoms Checklist

| Category | Symptoms | Possible causes |
|---|---|---|
| STOOL/ OUTPUT | **Narrow, ribbon-like** | Could be a sign of **stenosis** (a narrowing of the channel inside the intestine that the stool passes through). The narrowing might be up near the stoma opening, or further down inside. It can cause blockage and is often associated with Crohn's disease.<br><br>Other symptoms of stenosis can include cramps, burning or stinging inside the stoma while output is passing, diarrhea, increased gas, "explosive" stool, and a high-pitched sound when passing gas. |
| | **Too hard** | May be a result of medication (such as pain meds) or a lack of water, insoluble fiber, and/or magnesium in the diet. |
| | **Too soft** | If this only happens occasionally, it's probably something you ate ... or didn't eat (like enough fiber). If it's chronic, it could be a sign of an underlying medical condition. |
| | **Change in color** | If it's bright red, it could be fresh blood. If dark red or black, it could be dried blood or a side effect of iron supplements. But most often, it's something you ate. |
| | **Foamy** | If your output is foamy or consists of lots of little bubbles, this is often a sign of **gas**. It can also occur when you've gone a long time without eating. |

| Category | Symptoms | Possible causes |
|---|---|---|
| STOOL/ OUTPUT, cont'd. | Little or no output | Could be a **blockage** (more likely with ileostomies), or **constipation** (more likely with colostomies). Spurting liquid stool, a swollen stoma, feeling bloated, and dehydration symptoms are other symptoms of a blockage. Cramps are often present with both blockages and constipation. |

# Appendix C

# ILEOSTOMY BLOCKAGE GUIDE

The Emergency Blockage Card that appears on the following pages is provided by the United Ostomy Associations of America, Inc. (UOAA), a nonprofit organization that supports, empowers, and advocates for people who have had or who will have ostomy or continent diversion surgery.

On one side, the card provides information for treating an ileostomy blockage at home, and good advice on when to seek medical help.

The other side is designed to inform emergency room staff on how to treat ileostomy obstructions. If you suspect this is happening, it's important information to bring with you to the ER, as many non-specialized medical professionals have limited knowledge of ostomy management and treatment.

*This guide has been reprinted here with the kind permission of the UOAA.*

## APPENDIX C

### HOW TO TREAT ILEOSTOMY BLOCKAGE

**Symptoms:** Thin, clear liquid output with foul odor; cramping abdominal pain near the stoma; decrease in amount of or dark-colored urine, abdominal and stomal swelling.

**Step One: At Home**

1. Cut the opening of your pouch a little larger than normal because the stoma may swell.
2. If there is stomal output and you are not nauseated or vomiting, only consume liquids such as Coke, sports drinks, or tea.
3. Take a warm bath to relax the abdominal muscles.
4. Try several different body positions, such as a knee-chest position, as it might help move the blockage forward.
5. Massage the abdomen and the area around the stoma as this might increase the pressure behind the blockage and help it to "pop out." Most food blockages occur just below the stoma.

**Step Two: If you are still blocked, vomiting, or have no stomal output for several hours:**

1. Call your doctor or WOC/ET Nurse and report what is happening and what you tried at home to alleviate the problem. Your doctor or WOC/ET Nurse will give you instructions (ex., meet at the emergency room, come to the office). If you are told to go to the emergency room, the doctor or WOC/ET Nurse can call in orders for your care there.
2. If you cannot reach your WOC/ET Nurse or surgeon and there is **no output** from the stoma, go to the emergency room immediately.
3. **IMPORTANT:** TAKE THIS CARD WITH YOU TO THE EMERGENCY ROOM AND GIVE IT TO THE PHYSICIAN.
4. **IMPORTANT:** TAKE ALL OF YOUR POUCH SUPPLIES (eg., pouch, wafer, tail closure, skin barrier spray, irrigation sleeve, etc.)

© UOAA 2018

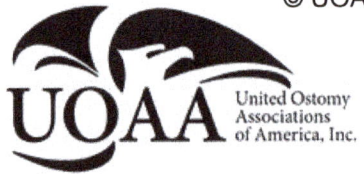

United Ostomy Associations of America
P.O. Box 525
Kennebunk, ME 04043
800-826-0826, www.ostomy.org

# EMERGENCY ROOM STAFF: ILEOSTOMY OBSTRUCTION

**Symptoms:** No stomal output; cramping abdominal pain; nausea and vomiting; abdominal distention, stomal edema, absent or faint bowel sounds.

1. Contact the patient's surgeon or WOC/ET Nurse to obtain history and request orders.
2. Pain medication should be initiated as indicated.
3. Start IV fluids (Lactated Ringer's Solution/Normal Saline) without delay.
4. Obtain flat abdominal x-ray or CT scan to rule out volvulus and determine the site/cause of the obstruction. Check for local blockage (peristomal hernia or stomal stenosis) via digital manipulation of the stoma lumen.
5. Evaluate fluid and electrolyte balance via appropriate laboratory studies.
6. If an **ileostomy lavage** is ordered, it should be performed by a surgeon or ostomy nurse using the following guidelines:

- Gently insert a lubricated, gloved finger into the lumen of the stoma. If a blockage is palpated, attempt to gently break it up with your finger.
- Attach a colostomy irrigation sleeve to the patient's two-piece pouching system. Many brands of pouching systems have Tupperware®-like flanges onto which the same size diameter irrigation sleeve can be attached. If the patient is not wearing a two-piece system, remove the one-piece system and attach a colostomy irrigation sleeve to an elastic belt and place it over the stoma.
- Working through the top of the colostomy irrigation sleeve, insert a lubricated catheter (#14–16 FR) into the lumen of the stoma until the blockage is reached. Do not force the catheter.
- **Note:** If it is possible to insert the catheter up to six inches, the blockage is likely caused by adhesions rather than a food bolus.
- Slowly instill 30–50 cc NS into the catheter using a bulb syringe. Remove the catheter and allow for returns into the irrigation sleeve. Repeat this procedure instilling 30–50 ccs at a time until the blockage is resolved. This can take 1–2 hours.

7. Once the blockage has been resolved, a clean, drainable pouch system should be applied. Because the stoma may be edematous, the opening in the pouch should be slightly larger than the stoma.

© UOAA 2018

# Index

1-piece system, 14
2-piece system, 15
Accordion flange, 25, 35, 144
Adhesion (scar tissue), 151
Adhesive pouches. *See* Self-adhesive pouches
Adhesive remover, 29, 43, 104
Adhesives. *See* Baseplate adhesives
Adynamic obstruction. *See* Paralytic ileus
Air travel, 74
Allergic dermatitis, 114, 151, 181
Anastomosis. *See* Reversal surgery
Ascending colon, 3
Bag liners, 30, 41, 85, 109, 145
Ballooning, 84, 104
Barbie butt, 141
Barrier. *See* Baseplate
Barrier paste. *See* stoma paste
Barrier rings, 17, 32, 105
Barrier sheets, 33, 105, 118
Barrier sprays, 34, 113
Barrier wipes. *See* Barrier sprays
Baseplate, 13, 17
Baseplate adhesives, 34, 118
Belly bands, 54
Bleeding, 10, 58, 121, 180
Blockages, 91, 96, 173, 183, 186
    UOAA emergency blockage card, 187
Blowouts, 106
Bowel resection, 152
Bulking agents, 90, 108
Burping (a pouch), 52, 86
Cecum, 3
Closed pouches, 23, 41
Colectomy, 152
Colon. *See* Large intestine
Colonoscopy, 142, 152
Colostomy, 3
Concave baseplates, 19, 128
Constipation, 87, 97, 168, 183, 186
Contact dermatitis, 112, 181
Convex baseplates, 19, 102, 120
Corticosteroids, 115
Crusting, 38, 113, 152
Cut-to-fit baseplates, 17, 101
Decision matrix
    1-piece vs 2-piece, 16
    adhesive vs mechanical coupling, 25
    drainable vs closed pouch, 23
    flat, convex, concave baseplate, 20

irrigation vs traditional system, 49
pre-cut, cut-to-fit, moldable, 18
regular vs extended wear, 22
regular vs floating flange, 26
Dehydration, 98
Deodorants, 82
Descending colon, 3, 46
Diarrhea, 97, 176
Diet
    constipation, 168
    diarrhea, 176
    food blockage, 173
    gas, 164
Digestive tract, 153
Disposal, 45
    as a houseguest, 73
    in hotels, 73
    in the workplace, 71
    when camping, 77
Double barrel stoma. *See* Mucous fistula
Drainable pouches, 22, 39
Dressing with an ostomy, 54, 79
Dynamic obstruction. *See* Mechanical blockage
Eating & drinking, 55
Electrolytes, 58, 98, 153
Emergency kit, 65
End ostomy, 153, 157
Enterostomal therapy nurse. *See* Stoma nurse
Excoriation, 153
Exercise, 87, 90, 94, 130, 133
Extended wear baseplates, 21
Fiber, 57, 89
Filters, 26, 84, 109
Fistula, 153
Flange (baseplate). *See* Baseplate
Flange (ring on baseplate), 24, 25
Flange extenders, 35, 78, 101, 119
Flat baseplates, 19
Flatulence, 71, *See* gas
Floating flange. *See* Accordion flange
Flush stoma, 102
Folliculitis, 182
Food tables, 163
Fungal infection, 115, 181
Gas, 51, 83, 164
Gentian violet, 116
Granulomas, 124, 154, 180, 182
Hair follicle inflammation, 117

Hernia belts, 131, 134, 146, 154
Hernias, 125, 154
   causes, 127
   complications, 128
   prevention, 130
   risk factors, 127
   treatment (non-surgical), 134
   treatment (surgical), 135
High output ileostomy, 141
Hospital visits, 68
   Emergency Blockage Card, 189
Hydration, 56
Ileostomy, 3
Ileostomy diarrhea. *See* High output ileostomy
Ileus, 92, *See* Paralytic ileus
Incarceration. *See* Hernias, complications
Incisional hernia. *See* Hernias
Inflammatory Bowel Disease (IBD), 155
Intimacy, 146
Irrigation, 2, 4, 46, 129, 155
Irritant dermatitis, 112, 155, 181
Ischemic ulcers, 184
Jackson Pratt drain, 137, 155
J-Pouch, 155
Laparoscopic surgery, 156
Large intestine, 2
Laxatives, 90, 95, 98
Leaks, 78, 100, 113
Loop ostomy, 141, 156
Loss of domain. *See* Hernias, complications
Low pressure adapter, 35, 144
Low residue diet, 57
Low-residue diet, 93
Lubricating deodorant, 35, 82, 109
Lumen, 156
Maceration, 181
Mechanical blockage, 92, 96, 157
Mechanical coupling, 24, 144
Mechanical irritation, 111
Medications, 58
Moldable baseplates, 18, 102
Mucocutaneous separation, 157, 180
Mucous fistula, 140, 141, 157
Mucus, 140, 141, 157, 180
Necrosis, 123, 158
Negative pressure wound therapy, 138, 158
Noises. *See* Stoma noises
Obstructions. *See* Blockages
Ostomy belts, 20, 118, 121
Ostomy scissors, 17, 36, 102
Ostomy wraps, 54
Pancaking, 19, 35, 104, 108

Paralytic ileus, 92, 158
Parastomal hernia. *See* Hernias
Pelvic tilt, 133
Peristalsis, 158
Pouch covers, 55
Pre-cut baseplates, 17
Pressure ulcers, 19, 112, 121, 182
Proctectomy, 158
Proctocolectomy, 158
Protective sheets. *See* Barrier sheets
Psoriasis, 182
Public bathrooms, 68
Pyoderma gangrenosum, 159, 182
Recovery from surgery, 5, 10, 55, 119, 131
Rectal stump, 159
Regular wear baseplates, 21
Retracted stoma, 102
Revision surgery, 159
Self-adhesive pouches, 86
Sex, 146
Short bowel syndrome, 159
Showering & bathing, 53
Sigmoid colon, 3, 46
Skin barrier sheets. *See* Barrier sheets
Skin barriers. *See* Barrier sprays
Skin irritations, 105, 110
Skin sealants. *See* Barrier sprays
Sleeping, 51
Small intestine, 2
Smells, 81
Smoking, 127, 131
Sphincter, 160
Stain removers, 107
Stenosis, 96, 160, 185
Stoma, 4, 9
   change in color, 123, 130, 184
   prolapse, 121, 129, 159, 183
   retracted or flush, 102, 120, 129, 159
   shape, 17, 119, 128
   size, 17, 119, 128
   swelling, 119, 120, 183
Stoma bridges, 36, 109
Stoma caps, 36, 80
Stoma collars, 37, 105
Stoma guards, 37, 54, 109
Stoma hats. *See* Stoma collars
Stoma noises, 71
Stoma nurse, 7, 161
Stoma paste, 31, 103
Stoma powder, 37, 113
Stoma protectors. *See* Stoma guards
Stool
   changing color, 145, 185

   foamy, 185
Strangulation. *See* Hernias, complications
Support groups, 7, 61
Swimming, 77
Symptoms
   blockage, 91
   constipation, 87
   diarrhea, 98
   skin irritation, 110
   symptoms checklist, 179
   yeast/fungal infection, 115
Templates (for cutting holes in baseplates), 17, 102

Toilet sprays, 82
Transit time, 4, 78, 141, 161
Transverse colon, 3
Travel, 72
Turtlenecking, 18
Vents, 85
Vitamins, 58
Wafer. *See* Baseplate
Water. *See* Hydration
Working, 69
Wound care nurse. *See* Stoma nurse
Wound vac, 137, 161
Yeast infection. See Fungal infection

www.ingramcontent.com/pod-product-compliance
Lightning Source LLC
Chambersburg PA
CBHW040222040426
42333CB00051B/3298